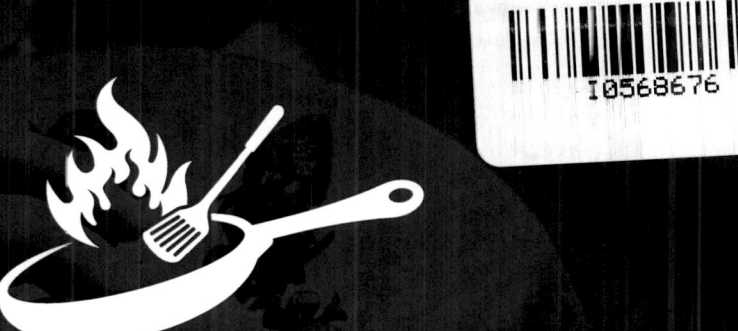

TrueJoy Living: A Sacred Relationship with Food

This isn't a book about new recipes — it's an invitation to return to yourself.
Food is energy, memory, and medicine — a bridge between body and soul.
Each dish, each ritual, each mindful bite is a way to root deeper into presence.
When you cook with intention, you create healing.
When you eat with gratitude, you awaken joy.
When you honor your body as a temple, you reconnect with your divine rhythm.

Through the six pillars of transformation — Ground, Awaken, Manifest,
Evolve, Conquer, and Embody — this book guides you to live
nourished, connected, and aligned.
Because nourishment is sacred.
Cooking is ceremony.
And every meal can be a moment of TrueJoy.

EAT WITH INTENTION.
LIVE IN ABUNDANCE.
EMBODY YOUR TRUE SELF.

This isn't just a cookbook — it's a journey.

Each recipe is designed as a ritual, pairing flavors with affirmations, ancient wisdom, and healing notes. From grounding soups and cleansing bowls to abundance cacao rituals, every meal helps you align body, mind, and spirit with your transformation.

Eat with presence. Cook with joy. Embody your best life.

90 Plant-Based Recipes Aligned with the 6 Pillars of the Breakthrough Blueprint with Optional Proteins & Cheeses by Pillar Supplements Guide

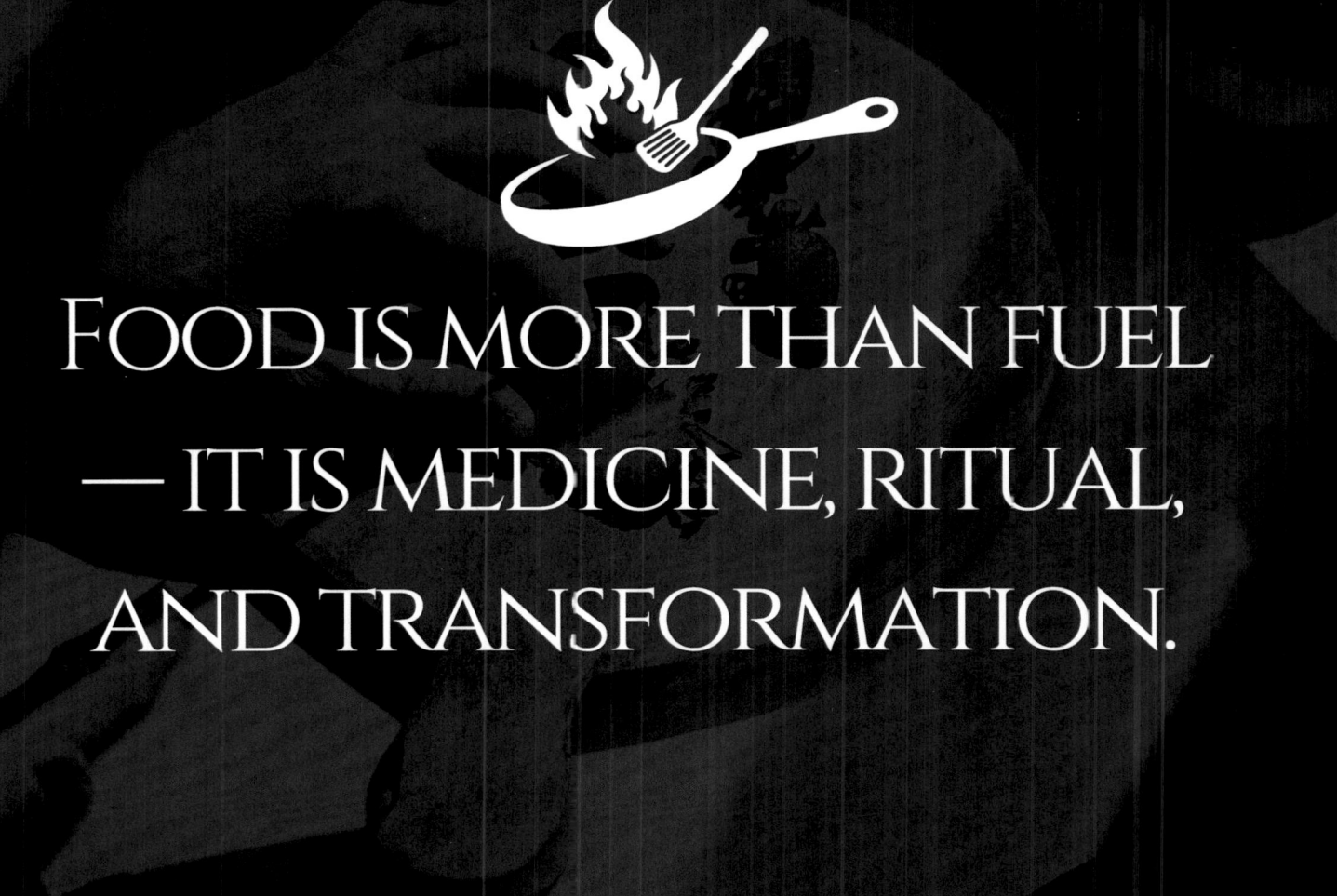

FOOD IS MORE THAN FUEL — IT IS MEDICINE, RITUAL, AND TRANSFORMATION.

Across history, cultures honored food as sacred:

Ayurveda (India): Food chosen for balance and healing.

Chinese Medicine: Seasonal eating aligned with nature's flow.

Indigenous Traditions: Meals as ceremony, gratitude, and connection.

Mediterranean & Greek Cultures: Food as vitality, abundance, and celebration.

In this cookbook, you'll find recipes for each pillar of the Breakthrough Blueprint. Each meal includes:

Mantra to align with the pillar's theme

Healing Note for body, mind, and spirit

Ancient Wisdom to connect with tradition

OPTIONAL PROTEINS & CHEESES

While the TrueJoy Living Master Recipe Book is rooted in plant-based meals, I also recognize that each person's journey with food is unique. Some may wish to include meat, poultry, seafood, or cheese as part of their lifestyle.

Rather than weaving these into each recipe, I've created this supplemental guide so that:
The recipes remain fully plant-based and accessible to everyone.
Readers who include animal-based foods still feel supported and guided.
Each addition aligns with the energetic qualities of the pillar it supports — grounding, awakening, manifesting, evolving, conquering, or embodying.

Whether you follow the book plant-based or adapt with these options, the intention remains the same: to eat with presence, honor food as medicine, and align nourishment with transformation.

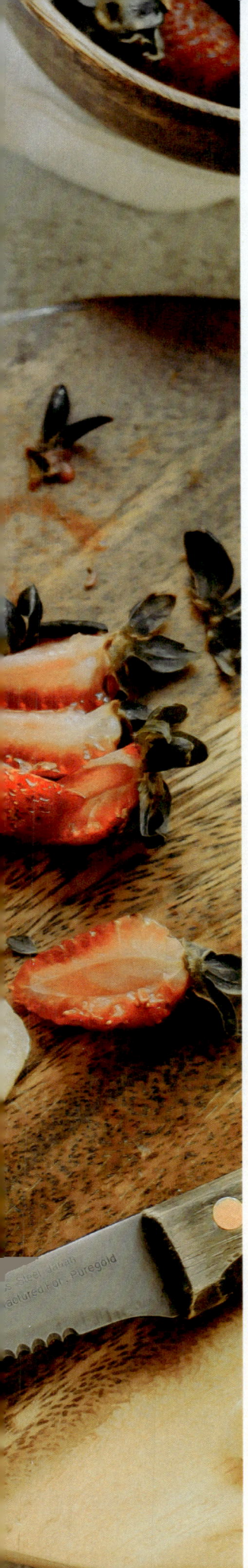

PILLAR 1
GROUND
ROOT, SAFETY, TRUST

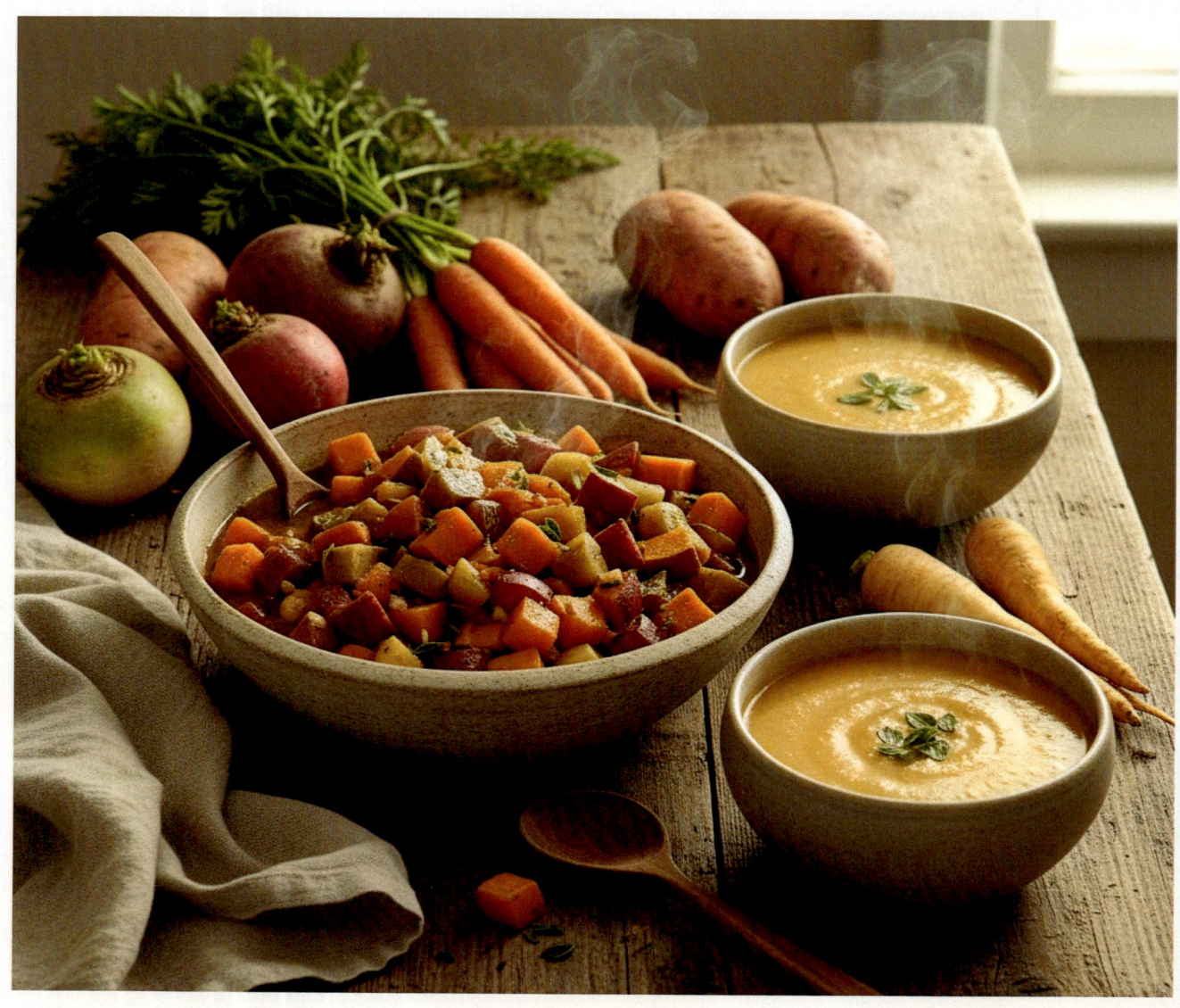

🍴 Optional Proteins & Cheeses

Ground – Root into Safety & Self-Trust

Mantra: "I root into nourishment and strength."
Healing Note: Protein-rich foods provide grounding energy and satiety.
Ancient Wisdom: Ancient hunters honored the animal spirit to anchor survival and stability.

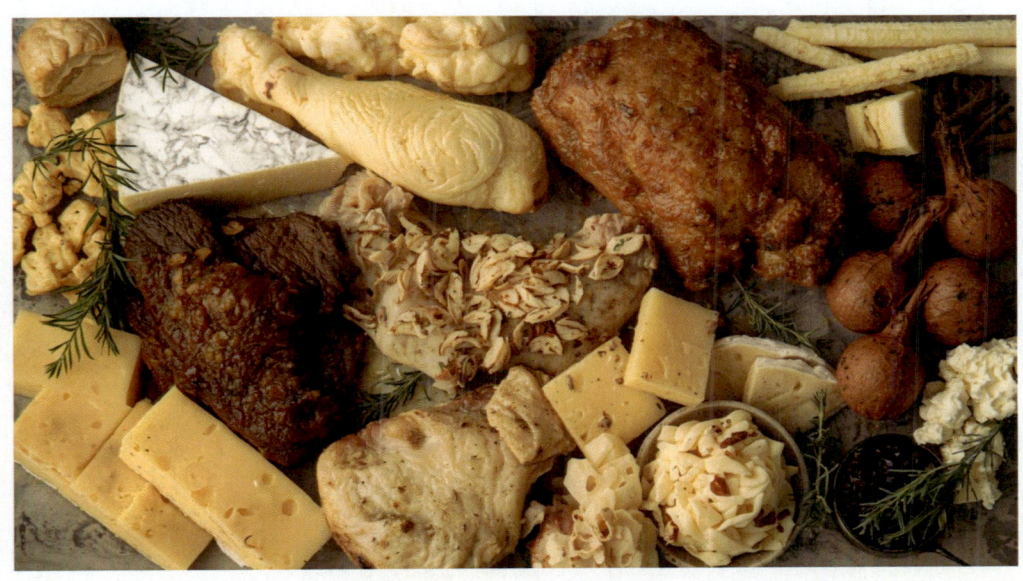

Meat (Beef/Bison): Slow-cooked for comfort.
Poultry (Chicken Thighs): Warming and steadying.
Seafood (Salmon): Omega-3s for calm focus.
Cheese (Cheddar/Goat): Pairs with roots, adds stability.

Sweet Potato Lentil Stew

Mantra: "I am safe. I am rooted."
Healing Note: Lentils balance blood sugar; sweet potatoes ground energy.
Ancient Wisdom: Lentils were among the first cultivated crops, symbolizing resilience.

INGREDIENTS: (4 SERVINGS)

- 1 tbsp olive oil
- 1 large onion, diced
- 3 cloves garlic, minced
- 2 carrots, diced
- 2 medium sweet potatoes, peeled & ½-inch cubes
- 1 cup red lentils, rinsed
- 6 cups vegetable broth (or water + bouillon)
- 1 tsp ground cumin
- ½ tsp ground turmeric
- ½–1 tsp salt, black pepper to taste
- (Optional) lemon wedge, chopped parsley

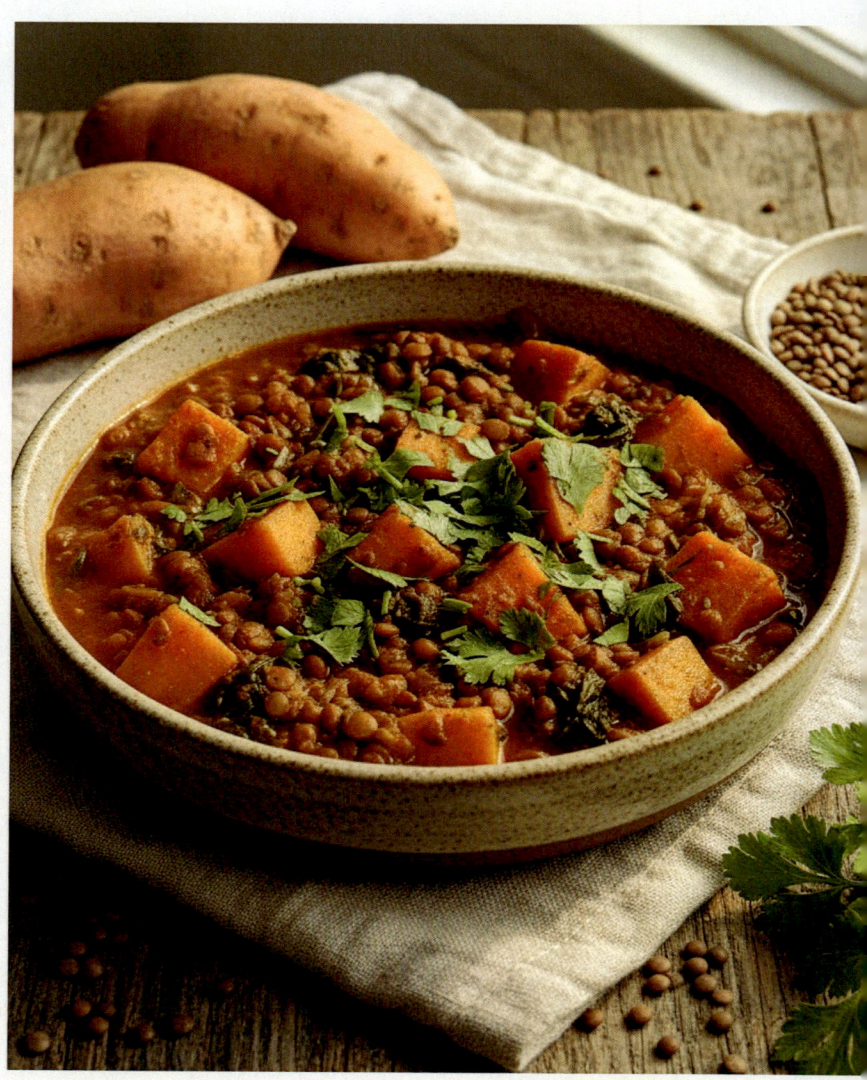

INSTRUCTIONS:

- Heat a large pot over medium. Add oil, onion, garlic, carrots; sauté 5 minutes until fragrant.
- Stir in sweet potatoes, lentils, broth, cumin, turmeric, salt & pepper.
- Bring to a boil, then reduce to a gentle simmer. Cover and cook 25–30 minutes until lentils and potatoes are tender.
- Taste and adjust seasoning. Finish with a squeeze of lemon and parsley if you like. Rest 5 minutes before serving.

Hearty Beet & Quinoa Bowl

Mantra: "I trust my path."

Healing Note: Quinoa is a complete protein; beets support circulation.

Ancient Wisdom: Quinoa was called "the mother grain" by the Inca.

INGREDIENTS: (2 SERVINGS)

- 1 cup cooked quinoa
- 2 medium beets, roasted, peeled, cubed*
- 2 cups baby spinach or mixed greens
- ½ avocado, sliced (optional)
- 2 tbsp pumpkin seeds or walnuts
- 1 tbsp olive oil
- Juice of ½ lemon
- Salt & pepper
- *To roast beets: Wrap whole beets in foil, bake at 400°F / 200°C for 40–60 minutes until tender. Cool, peel, cube.

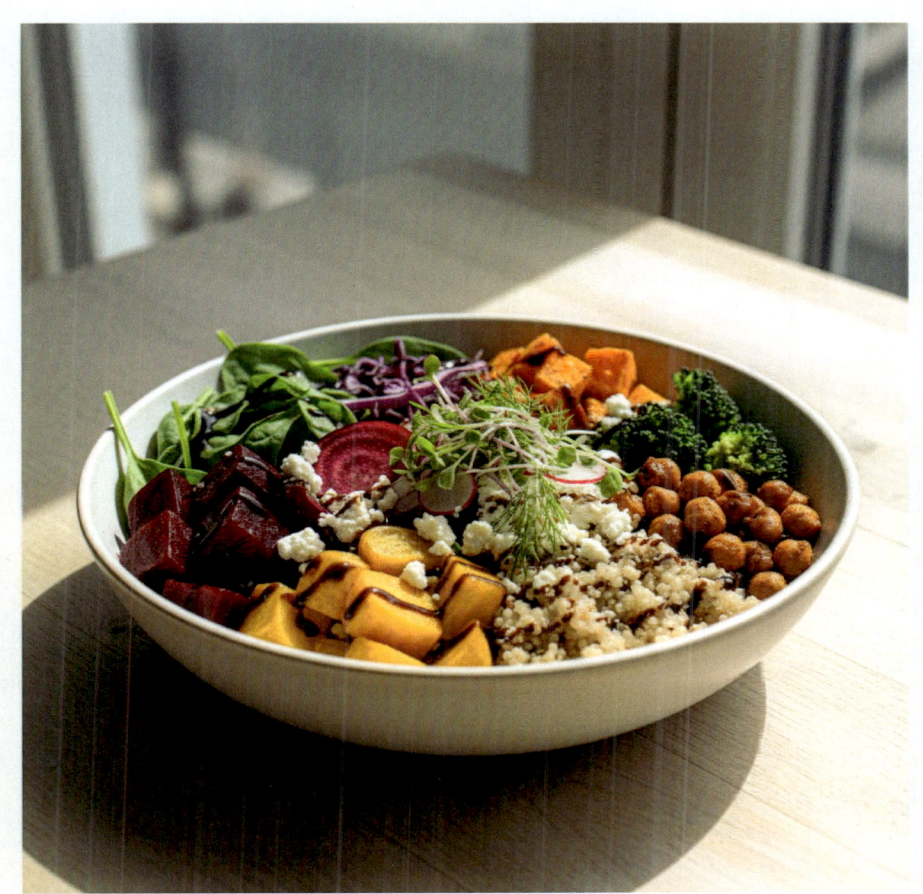

INSTRUCTIONS:

- Prepare quinoa and roast beets as above.
- Place spinach/greens in a bowl, top with quinoa and beets.
- Add avocado slices and seeds/nuts.
- Drizzle with olive oil, lemon, salt, and pepper. Serve warm or room temp.

Carrot Chickpea Nourish Bowl

Mantra: "I honor the Earth that nourishes me."
Healing Note: Chickpeas steady energy; carrots support clarity; seeds ground the body.
Ancient Wisdom: Chickpeas = sustenance in Middle East; sesame seeds = protection in Mesopotamia.

INGREDIENTS: (2 SERVINGS)

- 2 cups mixed greens or spinach
- 1 cup cooked chickpeas (rinsed & drained if canned)
- 2 carrots, grated or ribboned
- ½ avocado, sliced (optional)
- 2 tbsp sunflower or pumpkin seeds
- Tahini Lemon Dressing
- 2 tbsp tahini
- Juice of 1 lemon
- 1 tsp maple syrup or honey (optional)
- 1 tsp garlic powder or ½ clove grated garlic
- 2–4 tbsp water, to thin
- Pinch salt & pepper

INSTRUCTIONS:

- Whisk dressing: tahini, lemon, sweetener, garlic, salt/pepper; add water until pourable.
- Assemble bowls with greens, chickpeas, carrots, avocado.
- Sprinkle seeds, drizzle dressing, serve immediately.

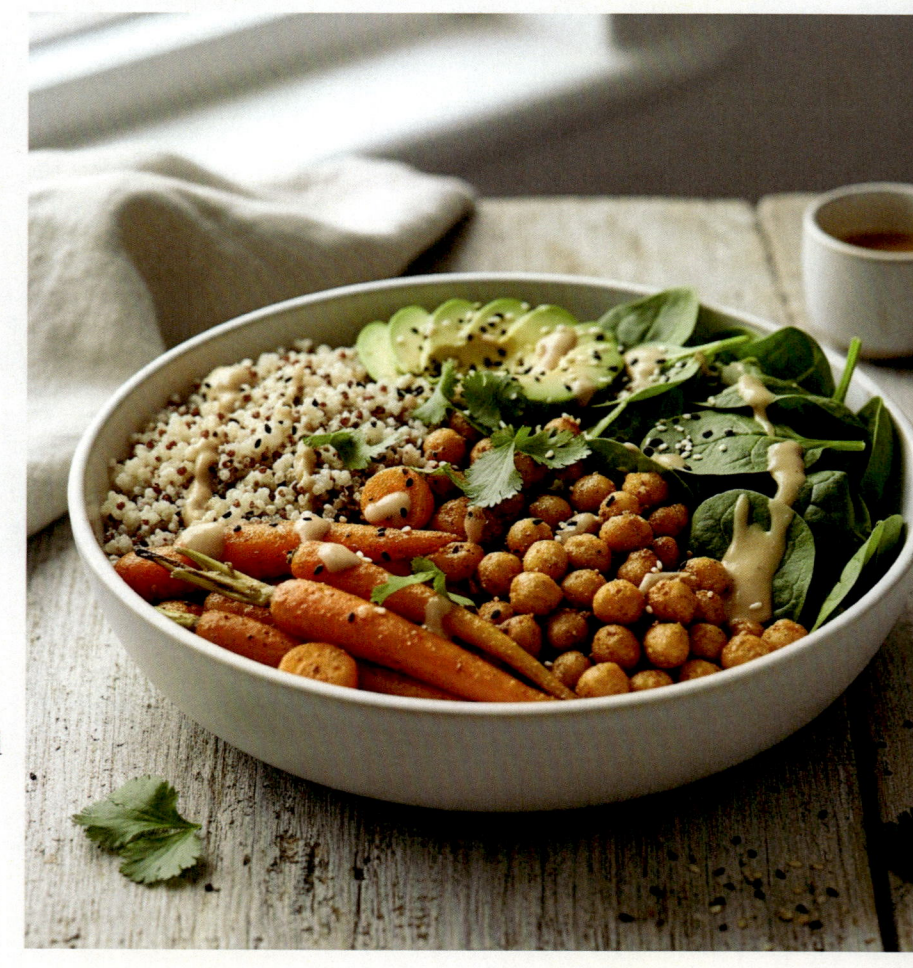

Southwest Stuffed Sweet Potatoes

Mantra: "I grow in trust each day."
Healing Note: Beans provide sustained energy; avocado adds nourishing fats.
Ancient Wisdom: Beans, corn, and squash — the "Three Sisters" — symbolized harmony in Indigenous cultures.

INGREDIENTS: (4 SERVINGS)

- 2 large sweet potatoes
- 1 cup cooked black beans (or 1 can, rinsed & drained)
- 1 cup corn (fresh, frozen, or canned)
- 1 red bell pepper, diced
- 1 small red onion, diced
- 1 tsp olive oil or avocado oil
- 1 tsp cumin
- ½ tsp smoked paprika
- ½ tsp chili powder
- Salt & pepper to taste
- ½ avocado, diced
- 2 tbsp fresh cilantro, chopped
- 1 lime (for juice)
- Optional toppings: vegan sour cream or Greek yogurt, salsa, jalapeños, pumpkin seeds

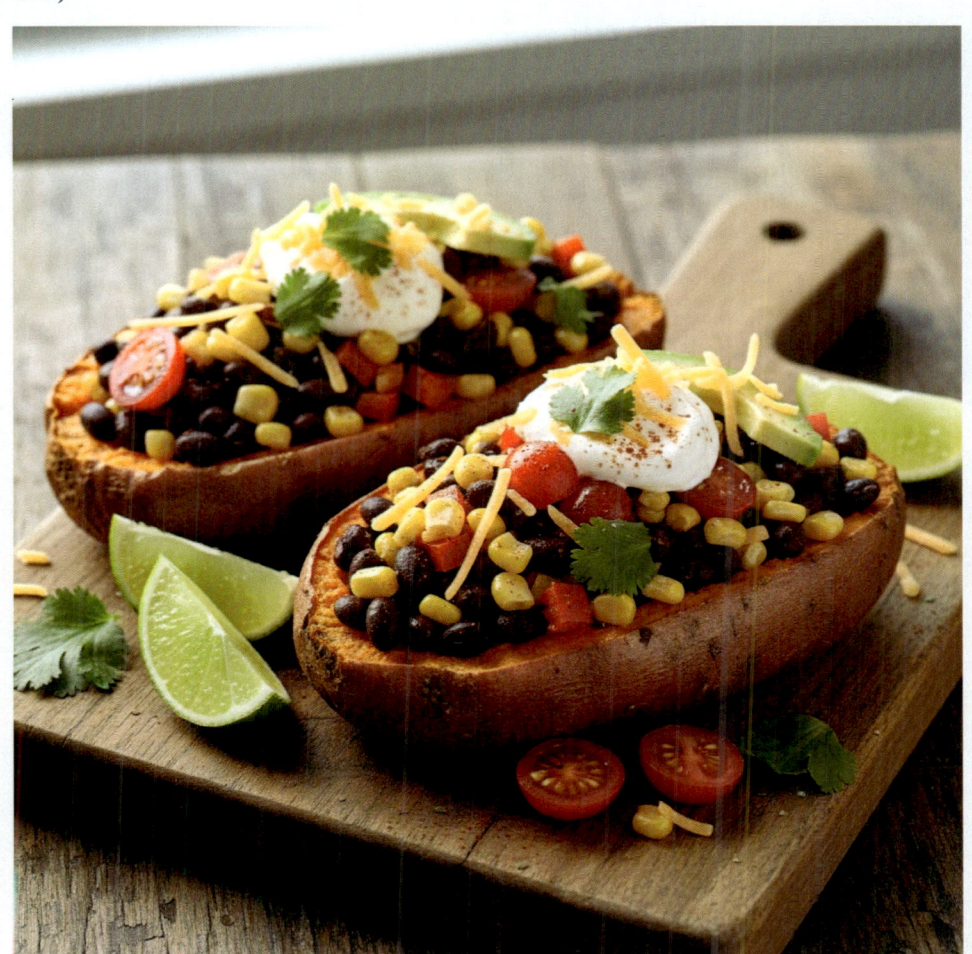

INSTRUCTIONS:

- Bake the Sweet Potatoes
- Preheat oven to 400°F (200°C).
- Wash sweet potatoes, poke a few holes with a fork.
- Place on a baking sheet and roast 45–50 minutes, until tender.
- Make the Filling- While sweet potatoes are baking, heat olive oil in a skillet.
- Sauté onion and bell pepper 3–4 minutes until softened.
- Add corn, black beans, cumin, paprika, chili powder, salt & pepper.
- Cook another 5 minutes, stirring until warmed through.

Assemble

Slice sweet potatoes open lengthwise and fluff with a fork. Spoon the bean & veggie mixture inside.
Top with avocado, cilantro, and a squeeze of lime.
Optional Add-ons
Drizzle with salsa or cashew-lime crema.
Sprinkle pumpkin seeds for crunch.

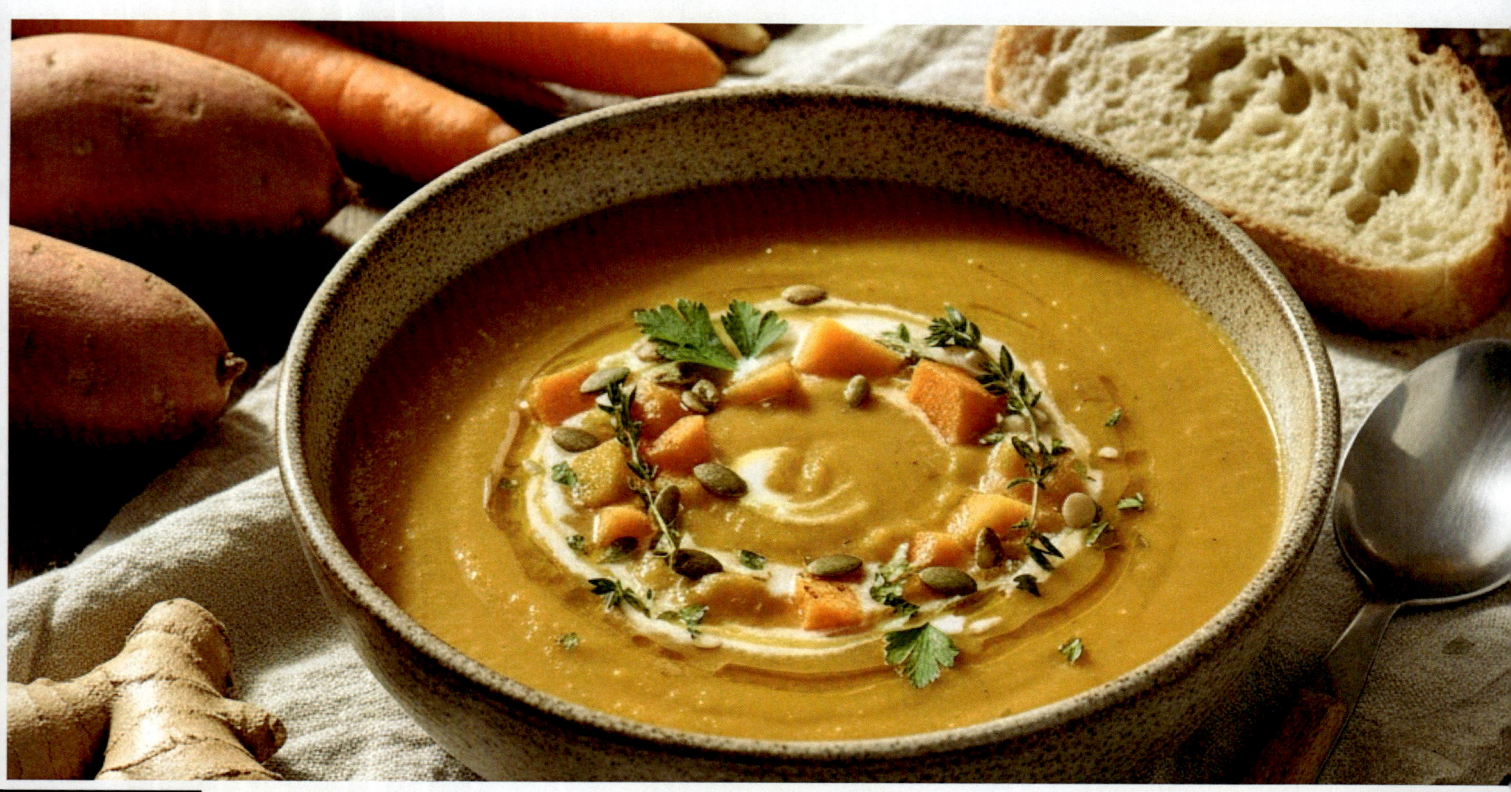

Golden Root Vegetable Soup

MANTRA: "I AM ROOTED IN SAFETY."
HEALING NOTE: TURMERIC REDUCES INFLAMMATION;   ROOTS NOURISH AND GROUND.
ANCIENT WISDOM: ROOT VEGETABLES HAVE LONG SYMBOLIZED STABILITY DURING SEASONAL CHANGE AND COMMUNITY FEASTS.

INGREDIENTS: (4 SERVINGS)

- 1 tbsp olive oil
- 1 onion, diced
- 3 carrots, chopped
- 2 parsnips (or extra carrots), chopped
- 2 cloves garlic, minced
- 1 tsp grated ginger (or ½ tsp ground)
- 1 tsp turmeric
- 4 cups vegetable broth
- Salt & pepper
- (Optional) splash coconut milk

INSTRUCTIONS:

- Heat oil in a pot; sauté onion 3 minutes.
- Add carrots, parsnips, garlic; cook 4 minutes.
- Stir in ginger and turmeric; toast briefly.
- Pour in broth, season, and simmer 20 minutes until tender.
- Blend all or part for creaminess; add coconut milk if desired.

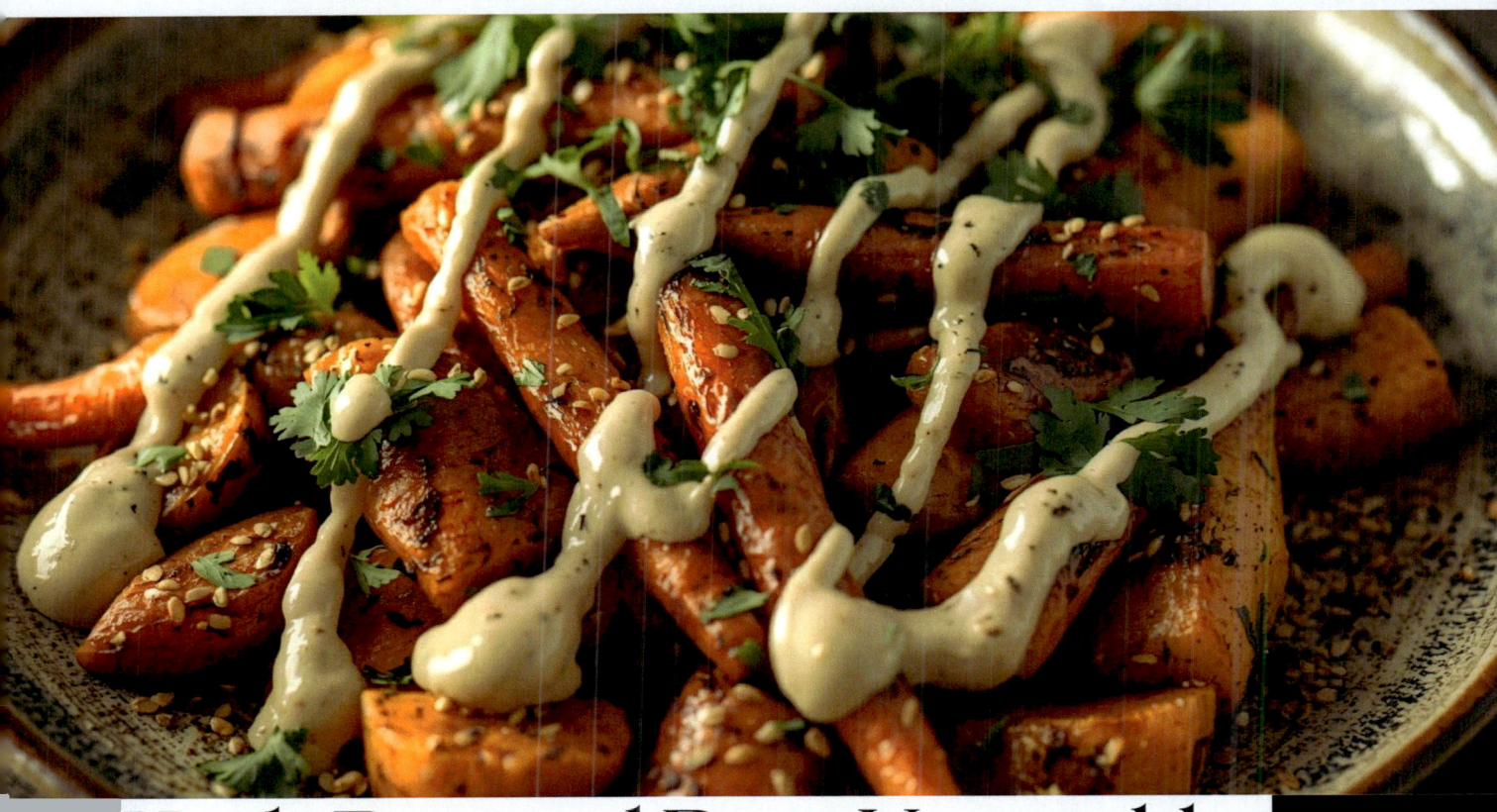

Herb-Roasted Root Vegetable Medley with Tahini Drizzle

MANTRA: "I AM ROOTED, STEADY, AND SAFE."
HEALING NOTE: ROOTS STABILIZE THE BODY'S ENERGY AND PROVIDE SLOW, GROUNDING NOURISHMENT.
ANCIENT WISDOM: ROASTED ROOTS WERE USED IN WINTER FEASTS FOR WARMTH AND RESILIENCE, SYMBOLIZING CONNECTION TO THE EARTH.

INGREDIENTS: (4 SERVINGS)

- 2 carrots, chopped
- 2 parsnips, chopped
- 1 sweet potato, cubed
- 1 golden beet, cubed
- 1 tbsp olive oil
- 1 tsp rosemary
- 1 tsp thyme
- Salt & pepper
- Sauce: 2 tbsp tahini + juice of ½ lemon + 1 tbsp warm water

INSTRUCTIONS:

- Preheat oven to 400°F.
- Toss all root veggies with oil, rosemary, thyme, salt, and pepper.
- Spread on a baking sheet and roast 30–35 minutes until golden and tender.
- Whisk tahini, lemon juice, and warm water into a drizzle.
- Plate roasted roots and finish with tahini sauce.

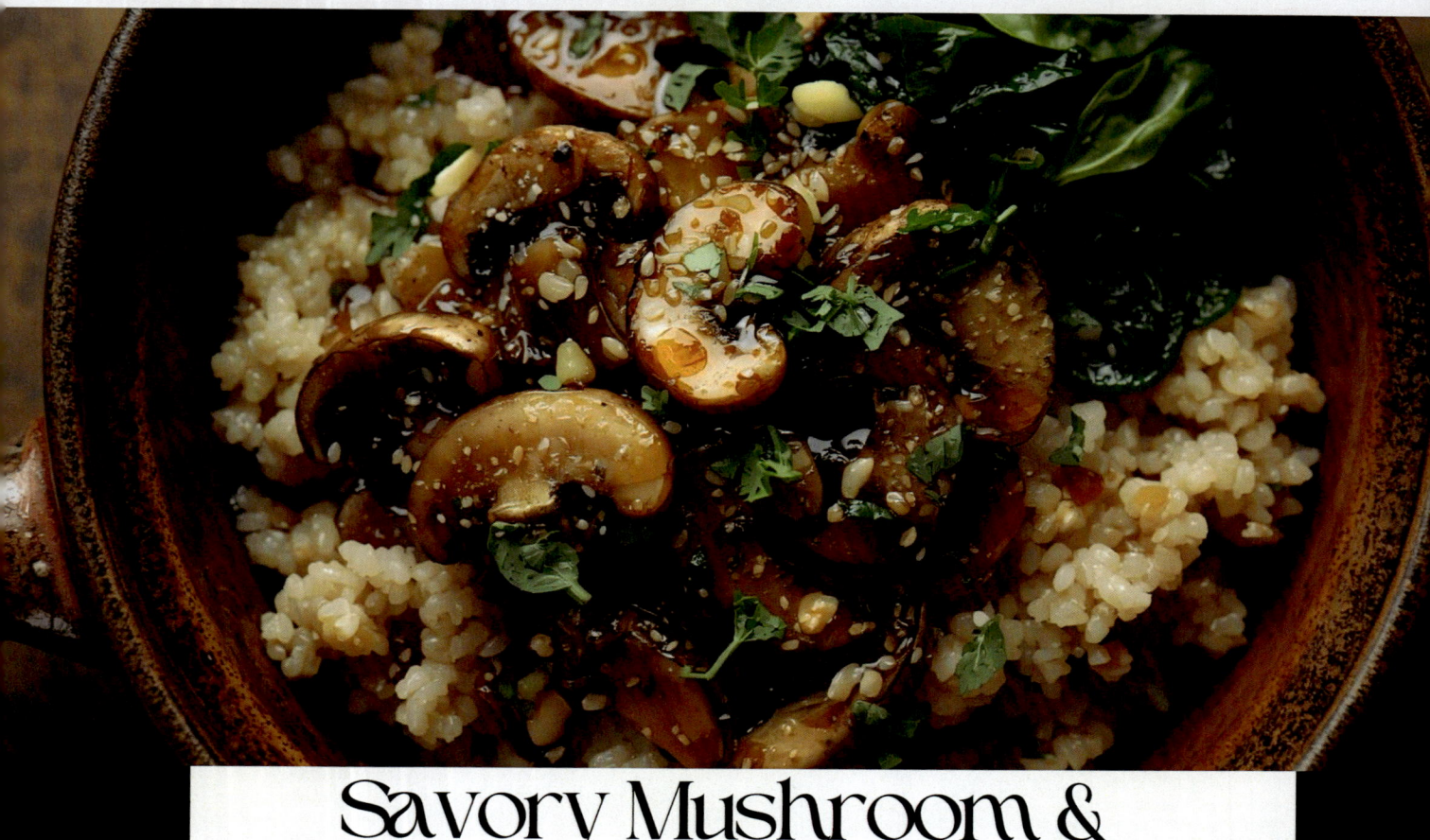

Savory Mushroom & Barley Bowl

MANTRA: "I TRUST MY PATH WITH GROUNDED STRENGTH."
HEALING NOTE: MUSHROOMS AND BARLEY PROMOTE GUT BALANCE AND IMMUNITY.
ANCIENT WISDOM: MUSHROOMS WERE REVERED BY ANCIENT CULTURES AS "EARTH'S MEDICINE,"
CONNECTING HUMANS TO THE WISDOM OF THE SOIL.

INGREDIENTS: (2 SERVINGS)

- 1 cup cooked barley
- 1 cup mushrooms, sliced
- 1 garlic clove, minced
- 1 tsp thyme
- 1 tbsp olive oil
- 1 tbsp tamari or soy sauce
- Handful of spinach

INSTRUCTIONS:

- Sauté mushrooms and garlic in olive oil until golden.
- Add thyme, tamari, and spinach; cook until wilted.
- Serve over barley for a hearty, earthy bowl.

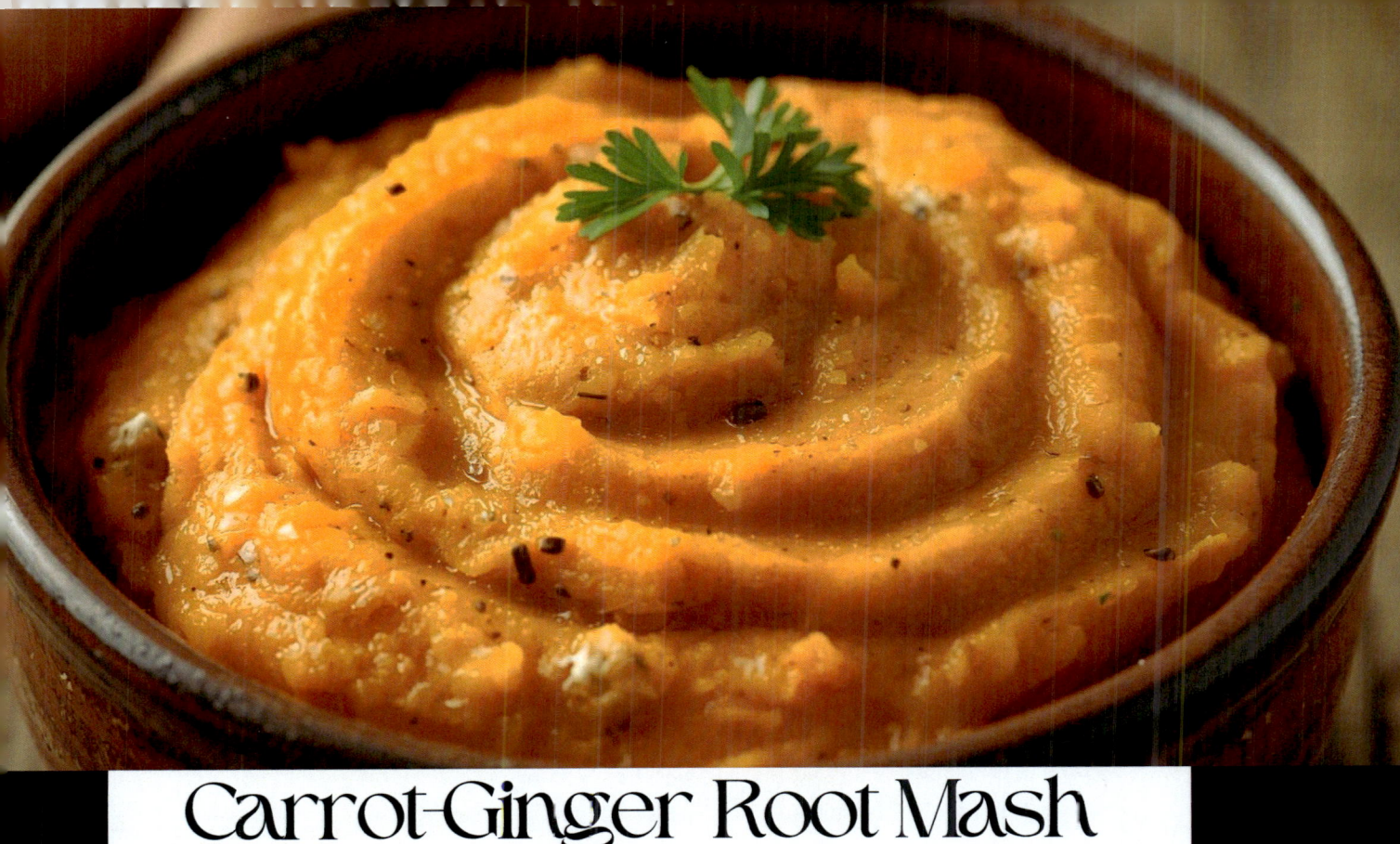

Carrot-Ginger Root Mash

MANTRA: "I AM SAFE, NOURISHED, AND AT PEACE."
HEALING NOTE: ROOT MASH SUPPORTS DIGESTION AND BOOSTS WARMTH THROUGH GINGER.
ANCIENT WISDOM: CARROTS AND PARSNIPS WERE SYMBOLS OF GROUNDING ENERGY AND
PROTECTION IN ANCIENT EUROPEAN WINTER RITUALS.

INGREDIENTS: (4 SERVINGS)

- 4 carrots, peeled and chopped
- 2 parsnips, peeled and chopped
- 1 tsp grated fresh ginger
- 1 tbsp coconut oil
- Salt to taste

INSTRUCTIONS:

- Boil carrots and parsnips until soft, about 15 minutes.
- Drain and mash with coconut oil and ginger.
- Season lightly with salt.

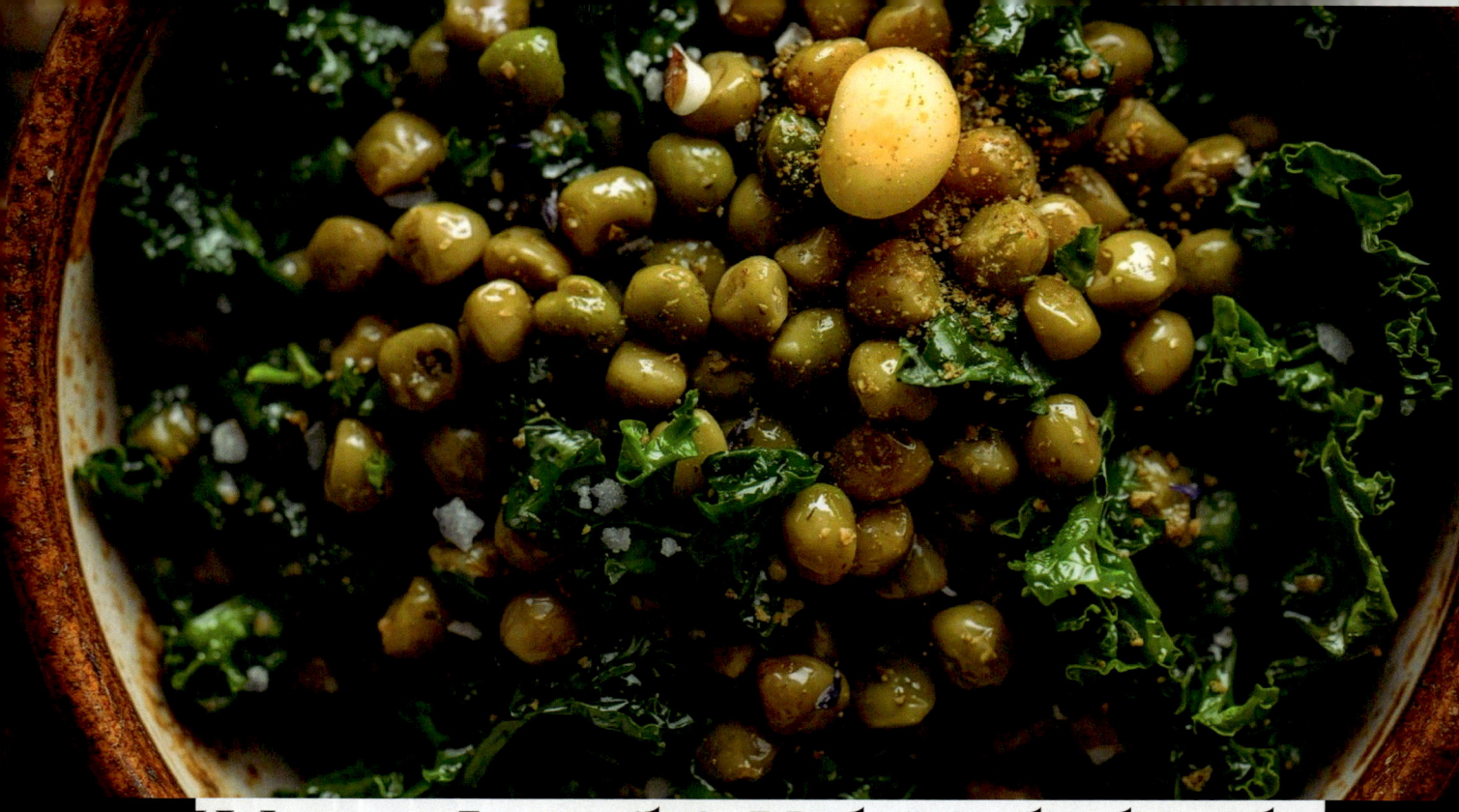

Warm Lentil & Kale Salad with Garlic Dressing

Mantra: "I honor my body's strength and roots."
Healing Note: Lentils ground the body; kale replenishes minerals and greens energy.
Ancient Wisdom: In ancient Greece, garlic and lentils were eaten to invoke vitality and protection.

INGREDIENTS: (2 SERVINGS)

- 1 cup cooked green lentils
- 2 cups chopped kale
- 1 tbsp olive oil
- 1 garlic clove, minced
- 1 tbsp apple cider vinegar
- Salt & pepper

INSTRUCTIONS:

- Heat olive oil, sauté garlic lightly.
- Add lentils and kale; toss until warmed and wilted.
- Drizzle with vinegar and season.

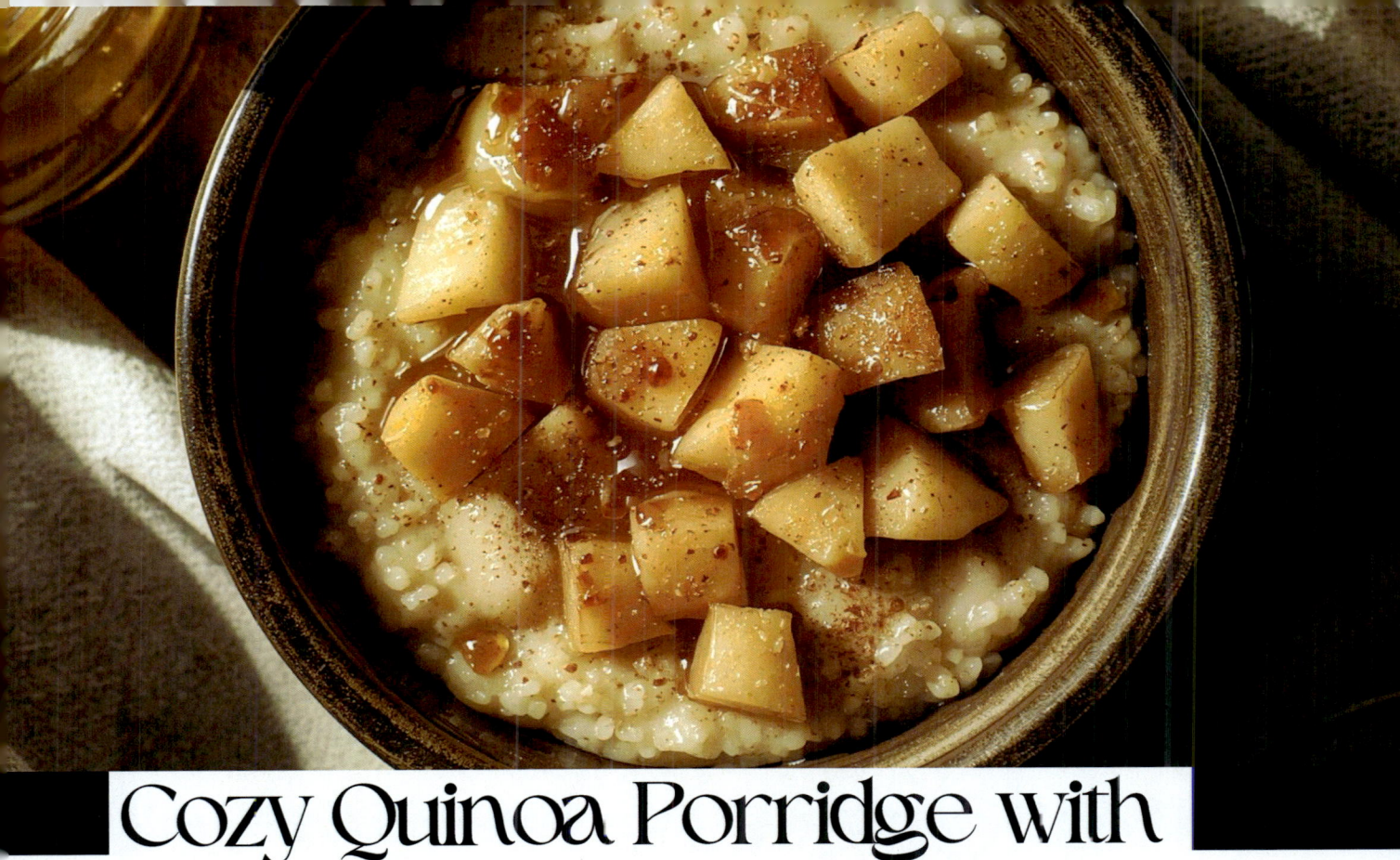

Cozy Quinoa Porridge with Spiced Apples

Mantra: "I am grounded in gratitude."

Healing Note: Quinoa provides complete protein; apples support digestion and emotional balance.

Ancient Wisdom: Warm grains were used in morning rituals as grounding energy for new beginnings.

INGREDIENTS: (2 SERVINGS)

- ½ cup quinoa
- 1 cup almond milk
- ½ cup water
- 1 apple, diced
- 1 tsp cinnamon
- 1 tbsp maple syrup
- 1 tsp coconut oil

INSTRUCTIONS:

- Simmer quinoa in milk and water for 15 minutes.
- Sauté apples in coconut oil and cinnamon until soft.
- Serve quinoa topped with apples and a drizzle of maple.

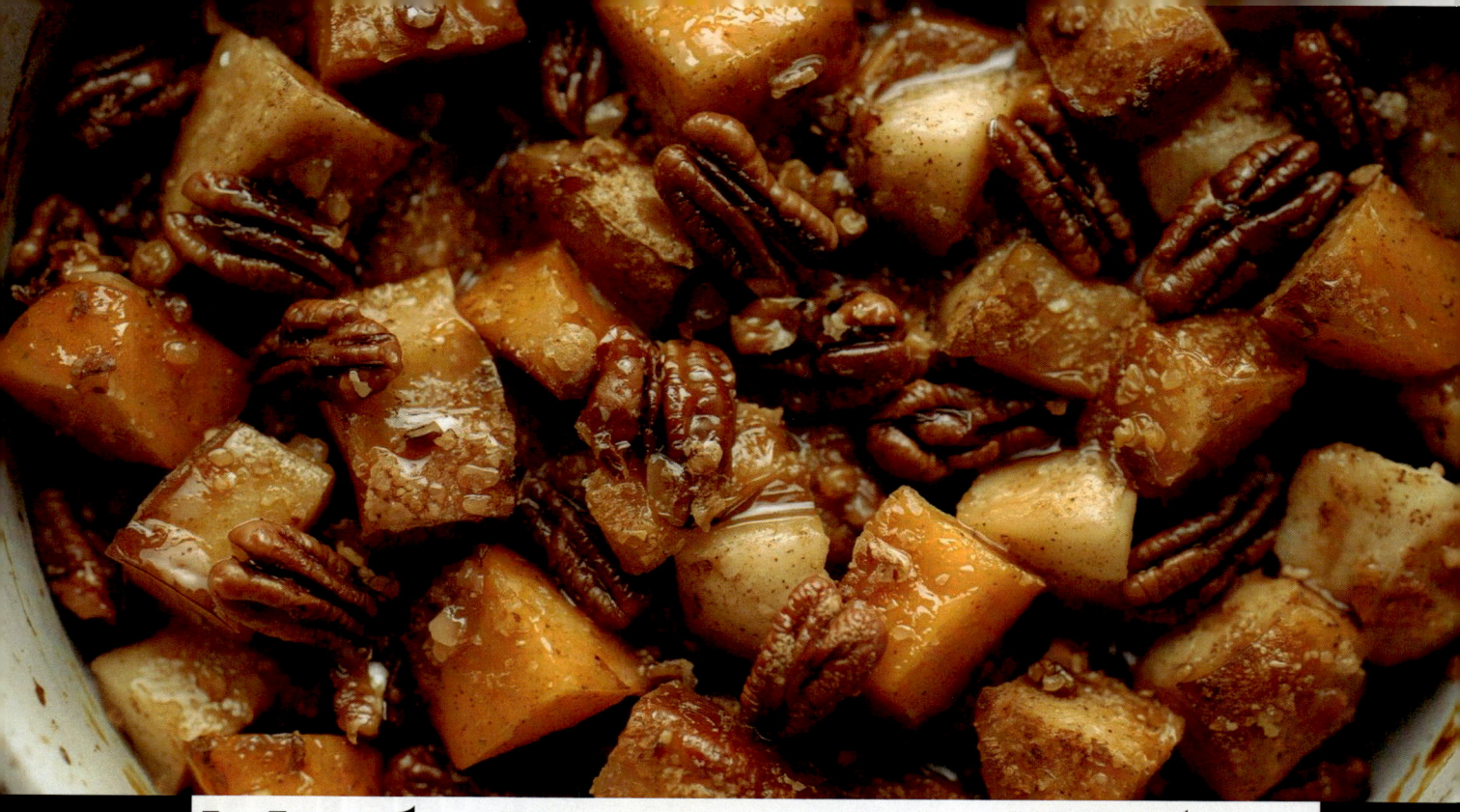

Maple Pecan Root Bake

Mantra: "I root into sweetness and stability."
Healing Note: Sweet potatoes and pecans provide warmth and comfort for emotional grounding.
Ancient Wisdom: Maple and tree nuts were ancient symbols of abundance and connection to the Earth's wisdom.

Ingredients: (4 servings)

- 2 sweet potatoes, cube
- 1 apple, sliced
- ¼ cup pecans
- 1 tbsp maple syrup
- 1 tbsp coconut oil
- 1 tsp cinnamon

Instructions:

- Preheat oven to 375°F
- Toss all ingredients and spread on a baking dish.
- Bake 30 minutes until golden and fragrant.

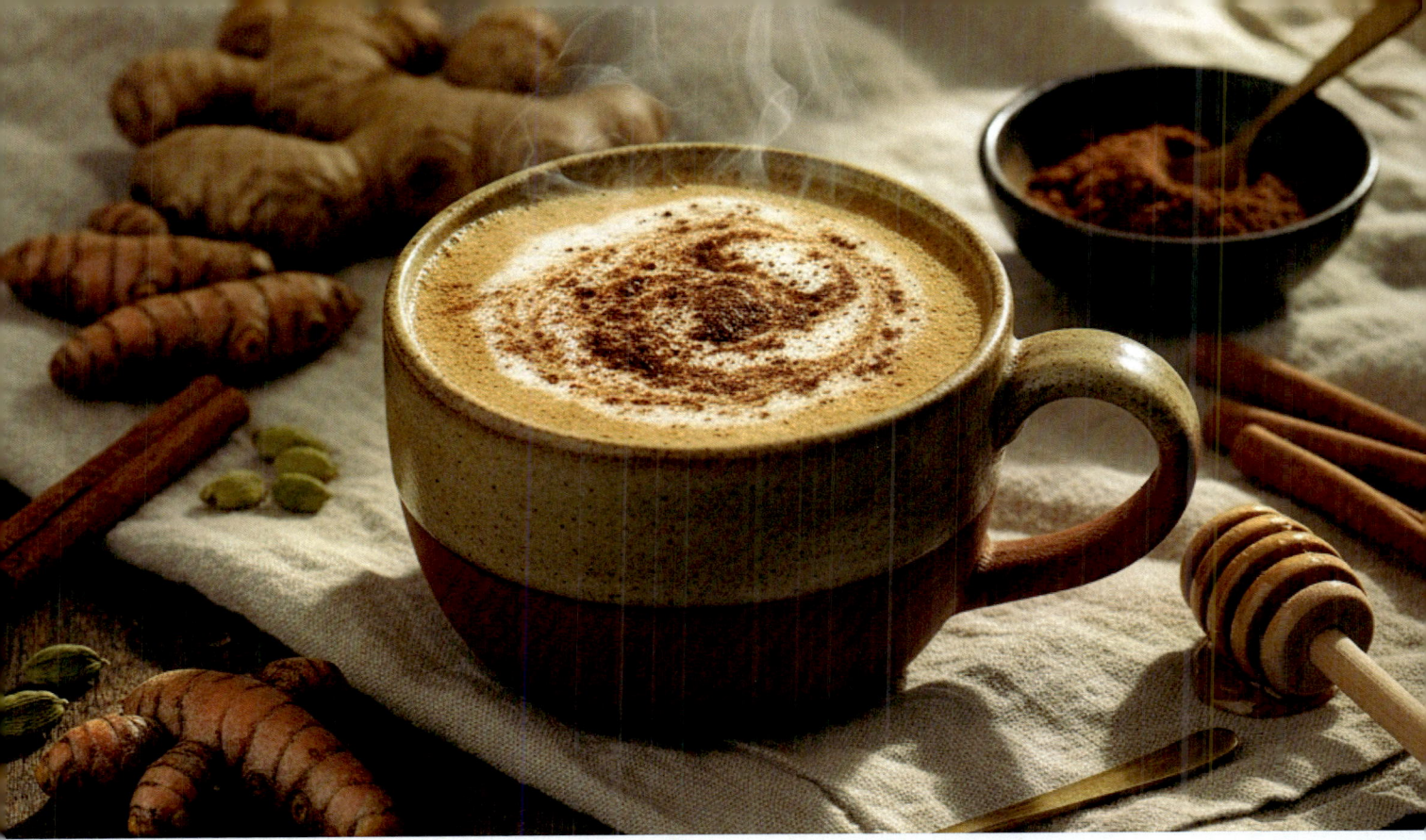

Cacao-Spiced Root Latte

MANTRA: "I AM STEADY. I AM STRONG."
HEALING NOTE: CACAO UPLIFTS THE HEART; CHICORY GROUNDS DIGESTION.
ANCIENT WISDOM: MAYANS USED CACAO AS A SACRED HEART MEDICINE.

INGREDIENTS: (2 MUGS)

- 1 cup strong brewed chicory root tea (or dandelion root/decaf coffee)
- 1 cup unsweetened almond or oat milk
- 1 tbsp raw cacao powder (or cocoa)
- ½ tsp cinnamon
- 1–2 tsp maple syrup (optional)
- Pinch sea salt

INSTRUCTIONS:

- Brew chicory root tea. Warm the milk in a small pot.
- Whisk cacao, cinnamon, maple, and salt into the warm milk.
- Divide tea between mugs, top with cacao milk, and sip slowly.

Spiced Chai Root Tea

Mantra: "I root into calm with every sip."
Healing Note: Warming spices support digestion.
Ancient Wisdom: Chai blends were used in Ayurveda for balance.

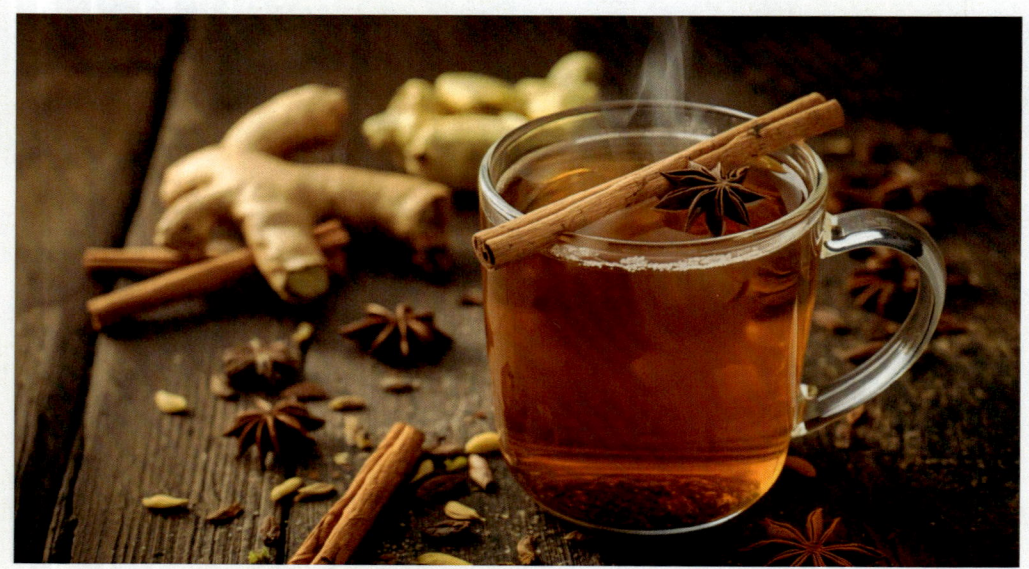

INGREDIENTS: (2 MUGS)

- 2 cups water
- 1 cinnamon stick
- 3 cardamom pods, crushed
- 2 slices fresh ginger
- 2 cloves
- 1 cup oat milk
- 1 tsp honey or maple (optional)

INSTRUCTIONS:

- Simmer spices in water 10 minute
- Add milk, simmer 5 minutes.
- Strain, sweeten, serve.

Golden Moon Milk with Ashwagandha & Lavender

MANTRA: "I RELEASE THE DAY AND ROOT IN PEACE."

HEALING NOTE: ABHWAGANDHA SOOTHES THE NERVOUS SYSTEM AND LOWERS STRESS, WHILE TURMERIC AND GINGER RELAX THE BODY AND SUPPORT NIGHTTIME RESTORATION. LAVENDER CALMS THE HEART AND MIND, GUIDING YOU GENTLY INTO DEEP, GROUNDED REST.

ANCIENT WISDOM: AYURVEDIC HEALERS HAVE LONG USED WARM SPICED MILK TONICS TO RESTORE BALANCE AND PREPARE FOR REST. IN MANY CULTURES, GOLDEN MILK SYMBOLIZED LIGHT RETURNING WITHIN — A SACRED REMINDER THAT PEACE IS FOUND BY TURNING INWARD BEFORE SLEEP.

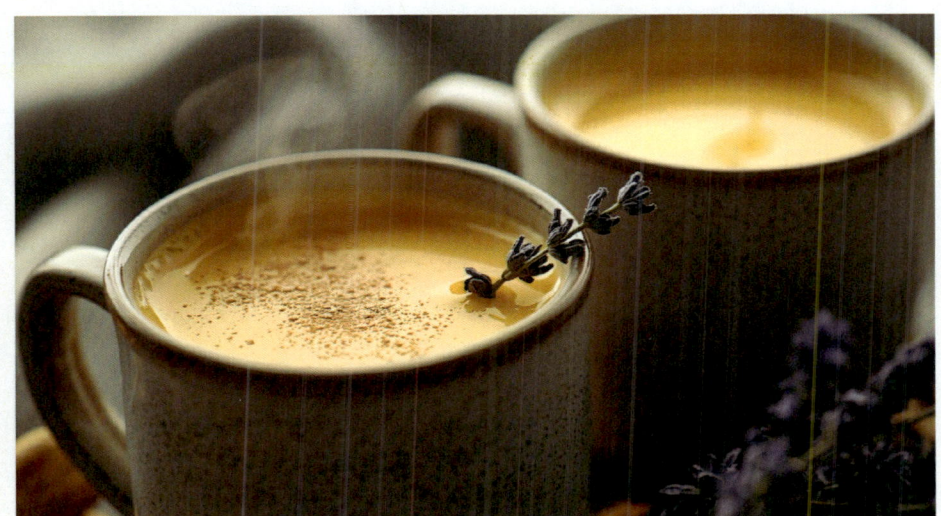

INGREDIENTS: (2 MUGS)

- 2 cups warm oat milk (or almond or coconut milk)
- ½ tsp turmeric powder
- ¼ tsp cinnamon
- ¼ tsp ground ginger
- ½ tsp ashwagandha powder (adaptogenic root for calm & restoration)
- ½ tsp dried culinary lavender (or 1 drop food-grade lavender extract)
- 1 tsp honey or maple syrup (optional)
- Pinch of nutmeg or cardamom (optional, for aroma & grounding)

INSTRUCTIONS:

- Warm milk gently in a saucepan over low heat — do not boil.
- Whisk in turmeric, cinnamon, ginger, and ashwagandha until smooth.
- Stir in lavender and let steep for 3–4 minutes, then strain (if using whole lavender).
- Sweeten with honey or maple syrup.
- Pour into your favorite mug, add a dusting of nutmeg, and sip slowly in stillness.

Baked Cinnamon Apples with Walnuts

MANTRA: "I SAVOR COMFORT AND SAFETY."
HEALING NOTE: APPLES SOOTHE, WALNUTS STRENGTHEN.
ANCIENT WISDOM: APPLES SYMBOLIZED HEALTH AND WHOLENESS IN FOLKLORE.

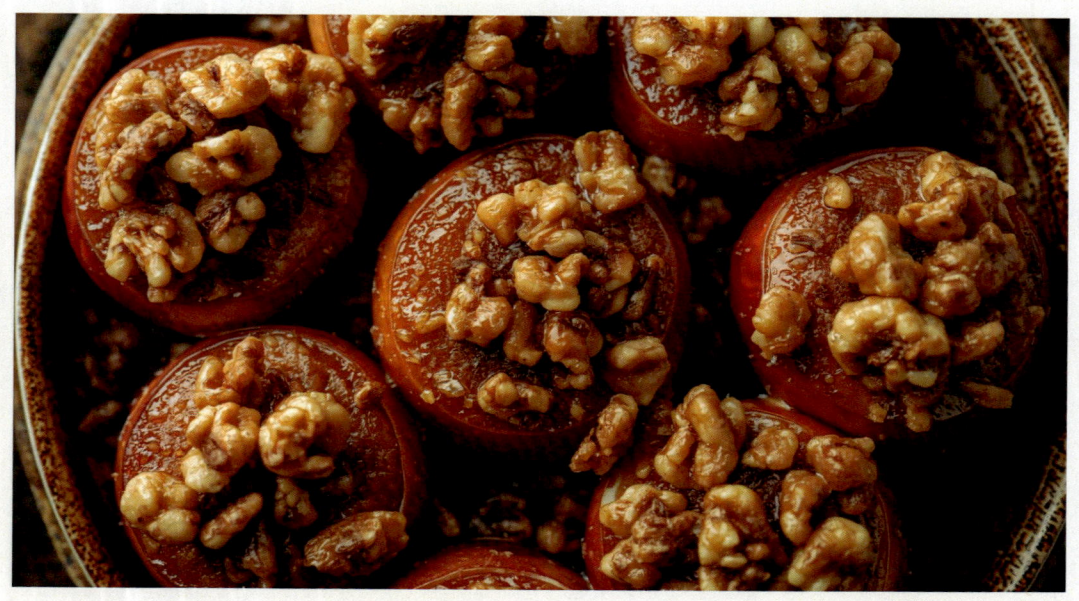

INGREDIENTS: (4 SERVINGS)
- 4 apples, cored
- ¼ cup rolled oats
- ¼ cup chopped walnuts
- 2 tbsp maple syrup
- 1 tsp cinnamon

INSTRUCTIONS:
- Mix oats, walnuts, maple, cinnamon.
- Stuff into apples.
- Bake at 375°F for 25 minutes until tender.

AWAKEN
Expand Presence & Energy

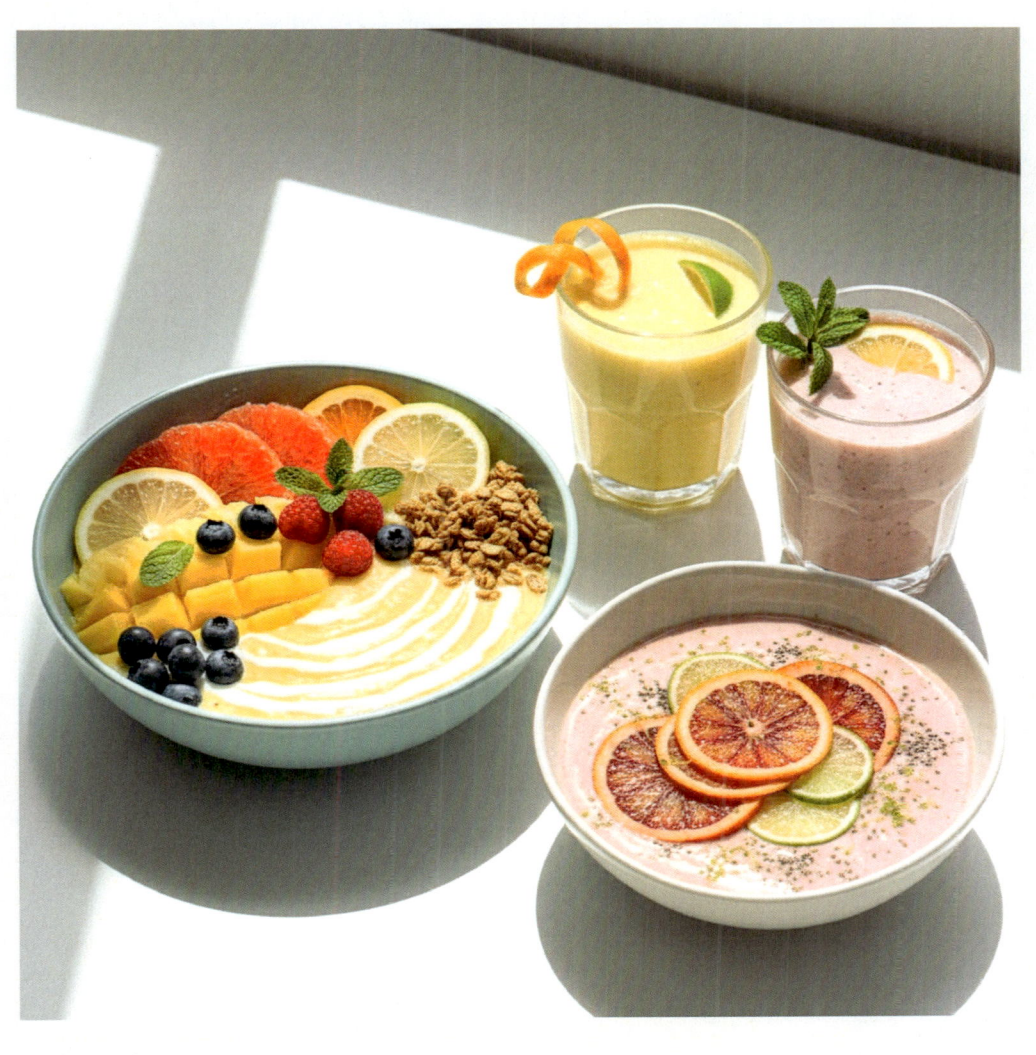

🍴 Optional Proteins & Cheeses

Awaken – Expand Energy & Intuition

Mantra: "I awaken my body with clarity."
Healing Note: Lean proteins enhance focus without weighing down energy.
Ancient Wisdom: Coastal cultures used seafood as a morning offering
to invoke freshness and vitality.

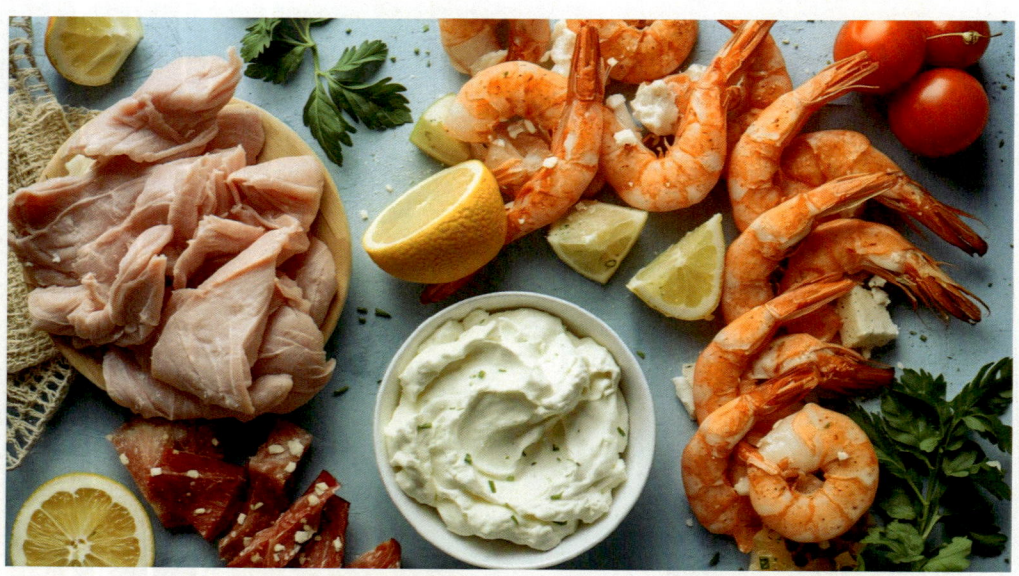

Meat (Turkey): Lean, energizing.
Poultry (Chicken Breast): Light, sustaining.
Seafood (Shrimp): Refreshing, vibrant with citrus.
Cheese (Feta/Ricotta): Bright and tangy.

Citrus & Berry Smoothie Bowl

MANTRA: "I AWAKEN WITH CLARITY."

HEALER'S NOTE: CITRUS + BERRIES LIFT ENERGY, ANTIOXIDANTS PROTECT THE BRAIN.

ANCIENT WISDOM: CITRUS WAS USED IN MEDITERRANEAN CLEANSING RITUALS.

INGREDIENTS: (2 SERVINGS)

- 2 cups frozen mixed berries
- 1 orange, peeled
- 1 banana
- 1 cup spinach
- 1 cup almond milk
- 2 tbsp flax or chia seeds
- Granola (for topping)

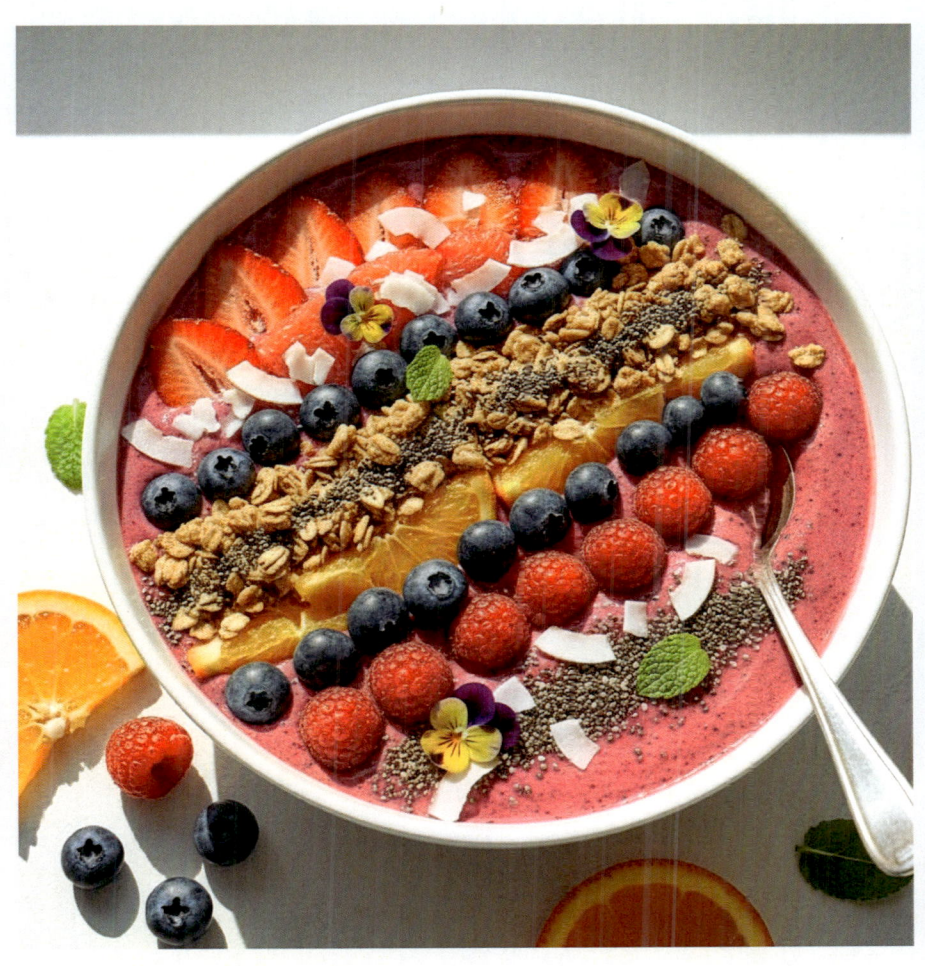

INSTRUCTIONS:

- Blend fruit, spinach, almond milk.
- Pour into bowls, top with seeds + granola.

Awaken Berry Oatmeal

Mantra: "I awaken with joy and sweetness."
Healing Note: Berries energize and brighten the body.
Ancient Wisdom: Berries were seen as celebratory foods, linked with vitality and spirit.

INGREDIENTS: (2 SERVINGS)

- 1 cup rolled oats
- 2 cups almond milk
- 1 cup mixed berries
- 1 tbsp flaxseeds
- 1 tsp maple syrup

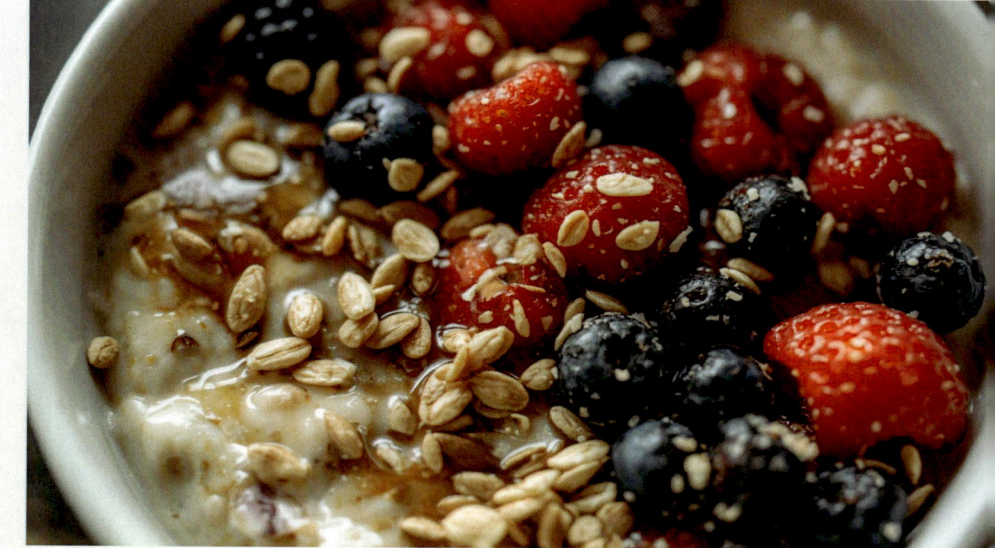

INSTRUCTIONS:

- Cook oats in almond milk.
- Stir in flaxseeds and maple syrup.
- Top with fresh berries.

Spring Awakening Salad

Mantra: "I choose energy and lightness."
Healer's Note: Radishes support liver detox; greens revitalize.
Ancient Wisdom: Radishes were sacred offerings in ancient Greece.

INGREDIENTS: (2 SERVINGS)

- 4 cups greens (spinach, arugula, kale)
- 1 cucumber, sliced
- 4 radishes, thinly sliced
- 1 avocado, cubed
- ¼ cup sunflower seeds
- Dressing: juice of 1 lemon, 2 tbsp olive oil, salt + pepper

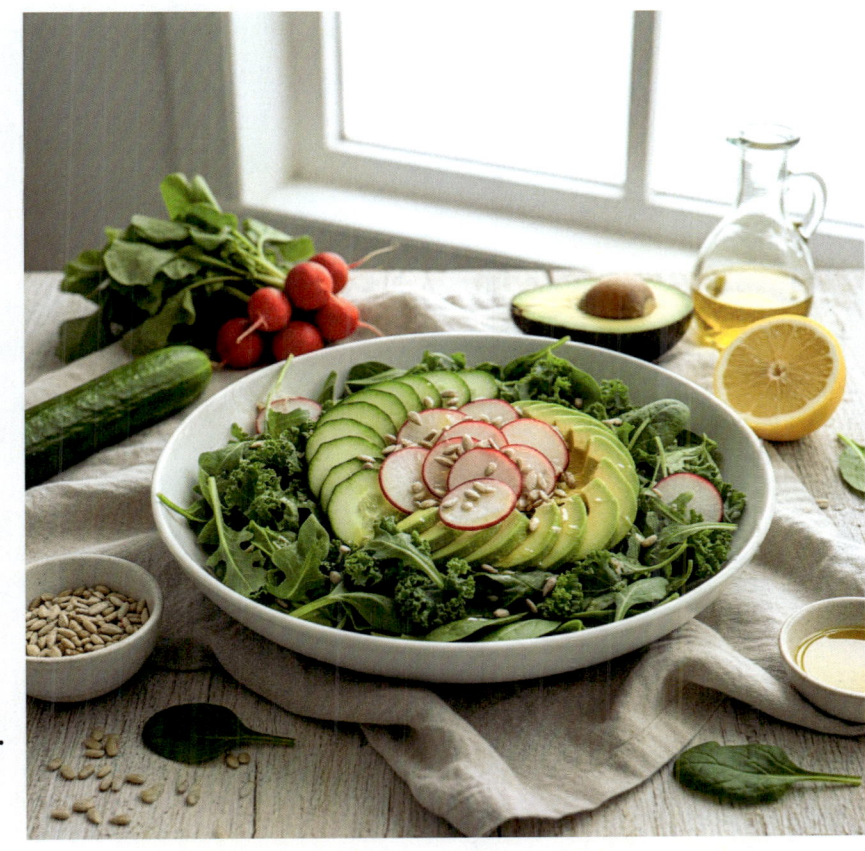

INSTRUCTIONS:

- Toss greens, cucumber, radishes, avocado.
- Whisk dressing, drizzle over salad.
- Top with sunflower seeds.

Sunshine Veggie Wraps with Citrus Dressing

Mantra: "I awaken with clarity and light."

Healing Note: Bright citrus and crunchy vegetables refresh energy and sharpen focus.

Ancient Wisdom: Citrus fruits were used in Mediterranean traditions to awaken the senses and cleanse stagnant energy.

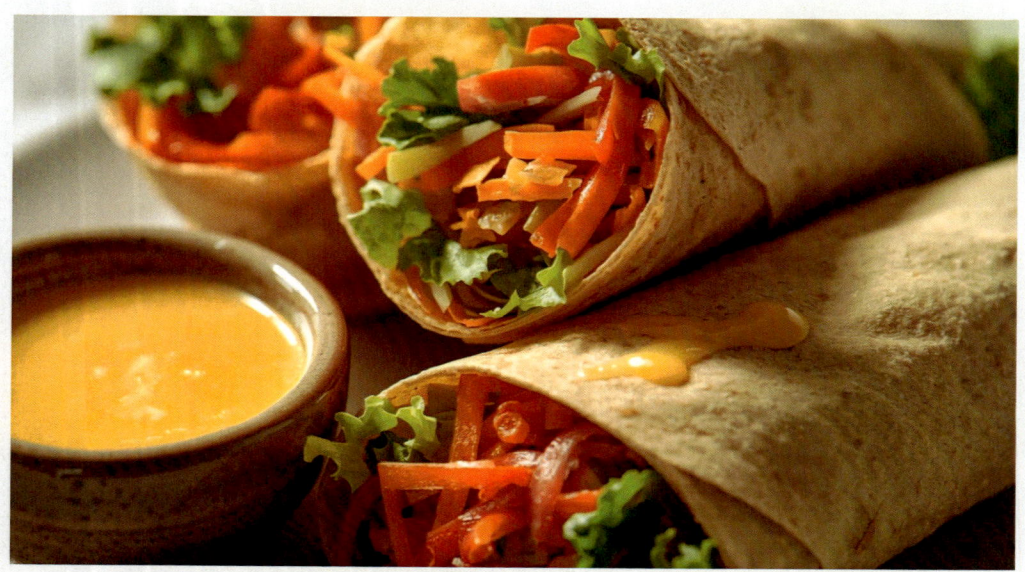

INGREDIENTS: (2 SERVINGS)

- 2 large whole-grain or collard green wraps
- 1 cup shredded carrots
- 1 cup cucumber strips
- ½ red bell pepper, thinly sliced
- ½ avocado, sliced
- ½ cup hummus
- 2 tbsp pumpkin seeds
- Citrus Dressing
- Juice of 1 orange
- 1 tbsp olive oil
- 1 tsp lemon zest
- Pinch of sea salt

INSTRUCTIONS:

- Spread hummus on each wrap.
- Layer carrots, cucumber, bell pepper, and avocado.
- Sprinkle with pumpkin seeds.
- Whisk dressing and drizzle lightly before rolling up.
- Slice in half and serve fresh.

Avocado Toast with Microgreens

Mantra: "I awaken to possibility with every bite."

Healing Note: Avocado fuels the brain with healthy fats.

Ancient Wisdom: Seeds and sprouts symbolized potential and growth.

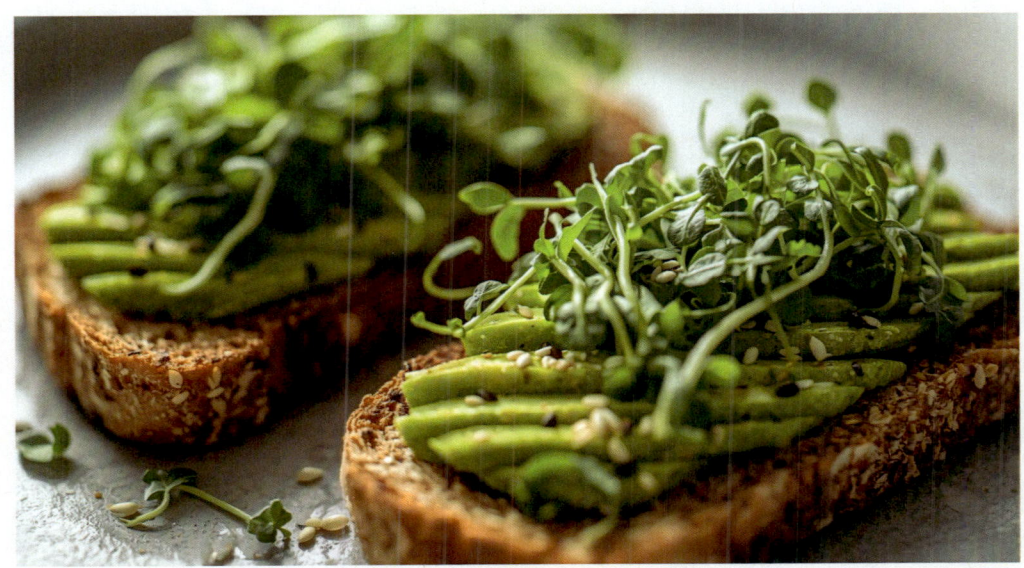

INGREDIENTS: (2 SERVINGS)

- 2 slices whole-grain bread
- 1 ripe avocado
- ½ cup microgreens
- 1 tsp sesame seeds
- Pinch of sea salt

INSTRUCTIONS:

- Toast bread slices.
- Mash avocado and spread evenly.
- Top with microgreens, sesame seeds, and sea salt.

Sunrise Veggie Buddha Bowl

Mantra: "I awaken with energy and clarity."
Healing Note: Citrus brightens; greens energize.
Ancient Wisdom: Lemon was used in Mediterranean rituals for purification.

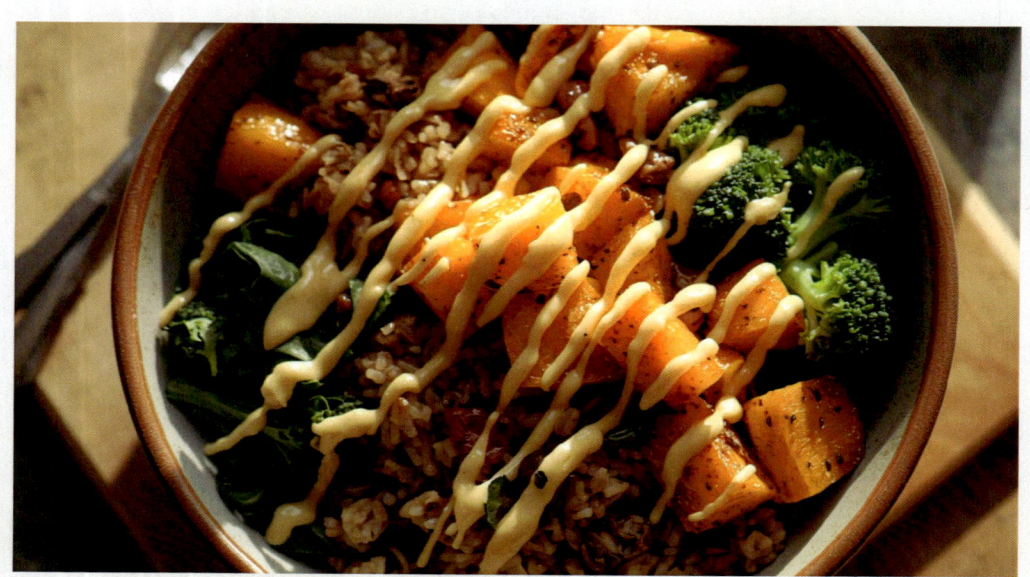

INGREDIENTS: (2 SERVINGS)

- 1 cup brown rice, cooked
- 1 cup sautéed greens
- 1 cup roasted squash cubes
- 1 cup steamed broccoli
- Dressing: 2 tbsp tahini + juice of 1 lemon

INSTRUCTIONS:

- Roast squash at 400°F for 20 minutes.
- Assemble rice, greens, squash, broccoli.
- Drizzle with lemon tahini dressing.

Rainbow Buddha Bowl

Mantra: "I open to new possibilities."
Healer's Note: Rainbow veggies deliver antioxidants + lift mood.
Ancient Wisdom: Rainbows have symbolized expansion across many cultures.

INGREDIENTS: (2 SERVINGS)

- 1 cup quinoa, cooked
- 1 cup chickpeas (roasted or canned)
- 1 cup shredded red cabbage
- 1 carrot, shredded
- 2 cups kale or spinach
- 1 avocado, sliced
- Dressing: 2 tbsp tahini, juice of 1 lemon, water to thin

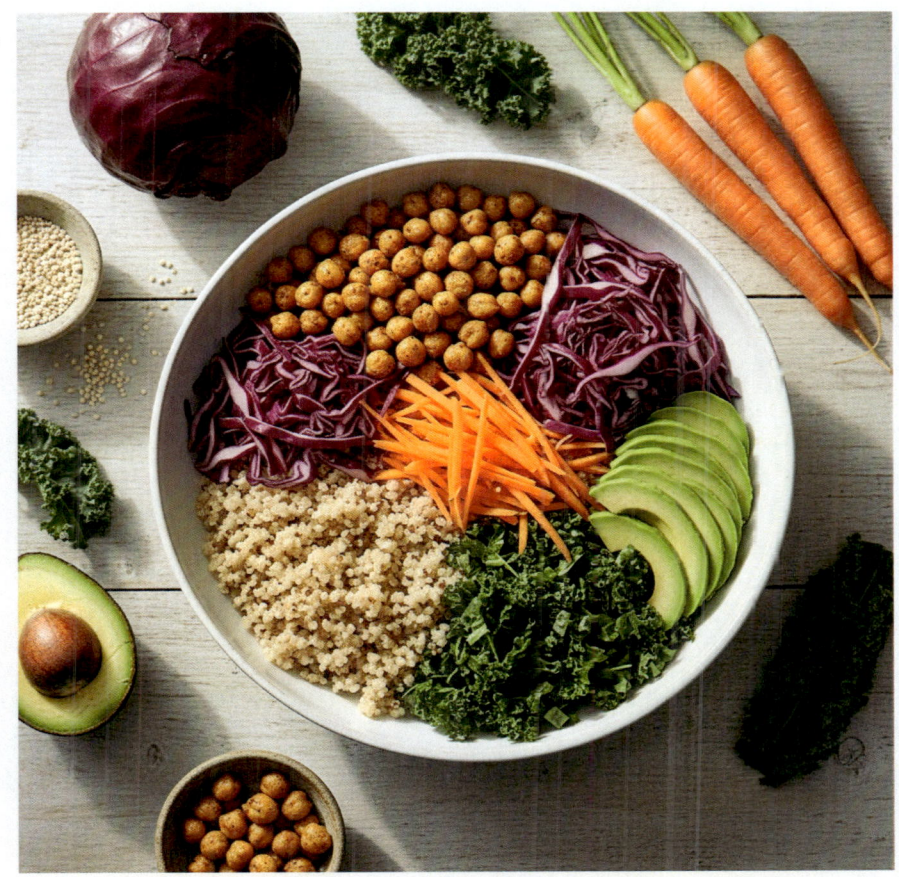

INSTRUCTIONS:

- Arrange quinoa, chickpeas, cabbage, carrot, greens, avocado.
- Whisk tahini + lemon, drizzle.

Zesty Quinoa & Citrus Salad

Mantra: "I awaken to fresh possibilities."
Healing Note: Citrus refreshes and boosts vitamin C; quinoa sustains energy.
Ancient Wisdom: Citrus fruits were long valued in the Mediterranean as symbols of vitality and renewal.

INGREDIENTS: (2 SERVINGS)

- 1 cup cooked quinoa, cooled
- 1 cup orange segments (or grapefruit mix)
- 1 cup baby spinach or arugula
- ½ cup cucumber, diced
- ¼ cup red onion, thinly sliced
- 2 tbsp pumpkin seeds
- Citrus Dressing
- Juice of 1 orange or lemon
- 2 tbsp olive oil
- 1 tsp honey or maple syrup
- Pinch salt & pepper

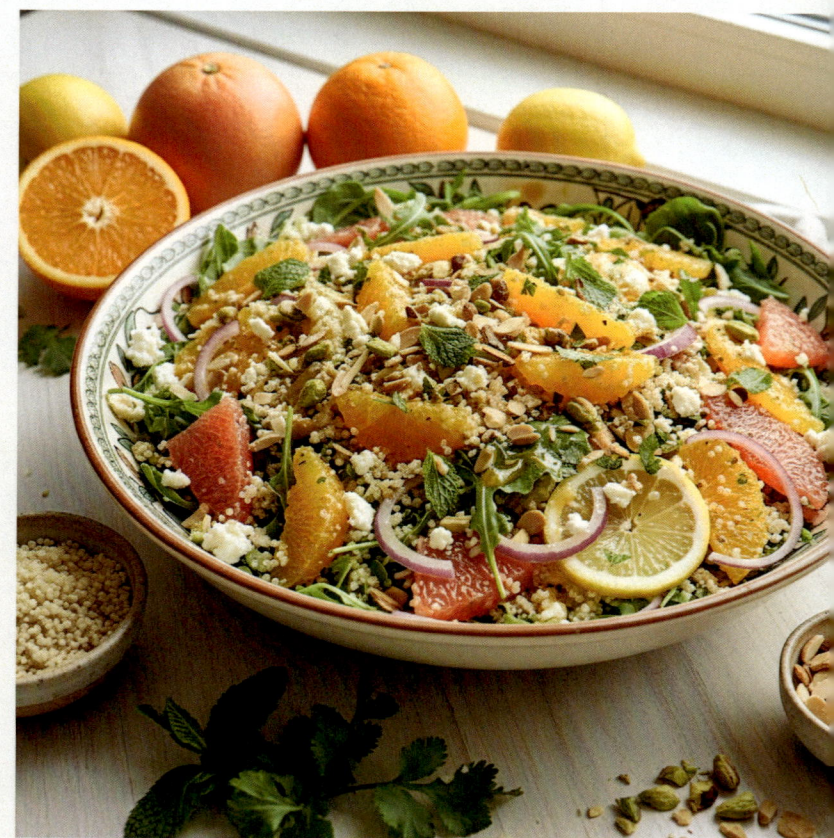

INSTRUCTIONS:

- In a large bowl, combine quinoa, citrus, greens, cucumber, and onion.
- Whisk dressing, pour over salad, toss gently.
- Sprinkle pumpkin seeds before serving.

Light Lemon-Ginger Lentil Soup

Mantra: "I am energized and clear."
Healing Note: Lentils give light protein; lemon and ginger uplift digestion and energy.
Ancient Wisdom: Ginger was prized in Ayurveda for awakening inner fire (agni); lemon symbolized cleansing and clarity.

INGREDIENTS: (2 SERVINGS)

- 1 tbsp olive oil
- 1 onion, diced
- 2 cloves garlic, minced
- 1 tsp fresh ginger, grated
- 1 cup red lentils, rinsed
- 5 cups vegetable broth
- Zest + juice of 1 lemon
- 2 cups baby spinach
- Salt & pepper to taste

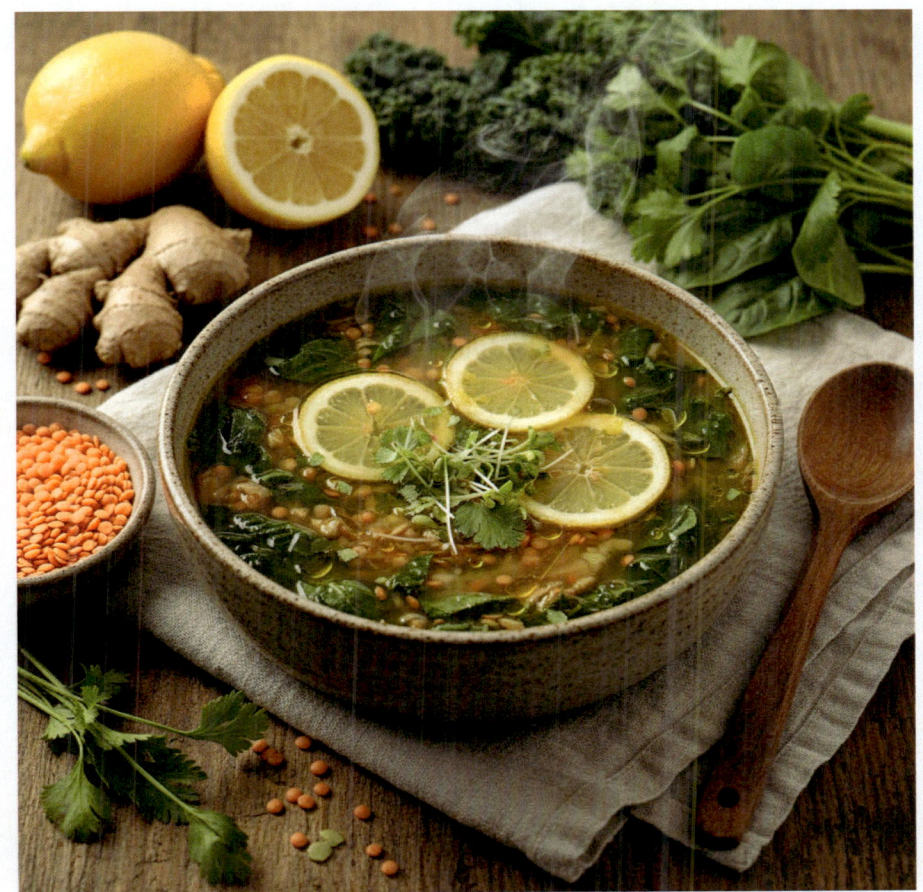

INSTRUCTIONS:

- Heat oil; sauté onion 4 minutes, add garlic and ginger 1 minute.
- Stir in lentils and broth, bring to boil, then simmer 20 minutes.
- Stir in lemon zest, juice, and spinach; season with salt/pepper.
- Serve warm with fresh herbs if desired.

Matcha Chia Pudding

Mantra: "My mind is clear and focused."
Healer's Note: Matcha sustains calm energy; chia seeds stabilize blood sugar.
Ancient Wisdom: Zen monks drank matcha to remain awake in meditation.

INGREDIENTS: (2 SERVINGS)

- 1 ½ cups almond milk
- ½ cup chia seeds
- 1 tbsp matcha powder
- 1 tsp vanilla extract
- 1–2 tbsp maple syrup
- ½ cup blueberries

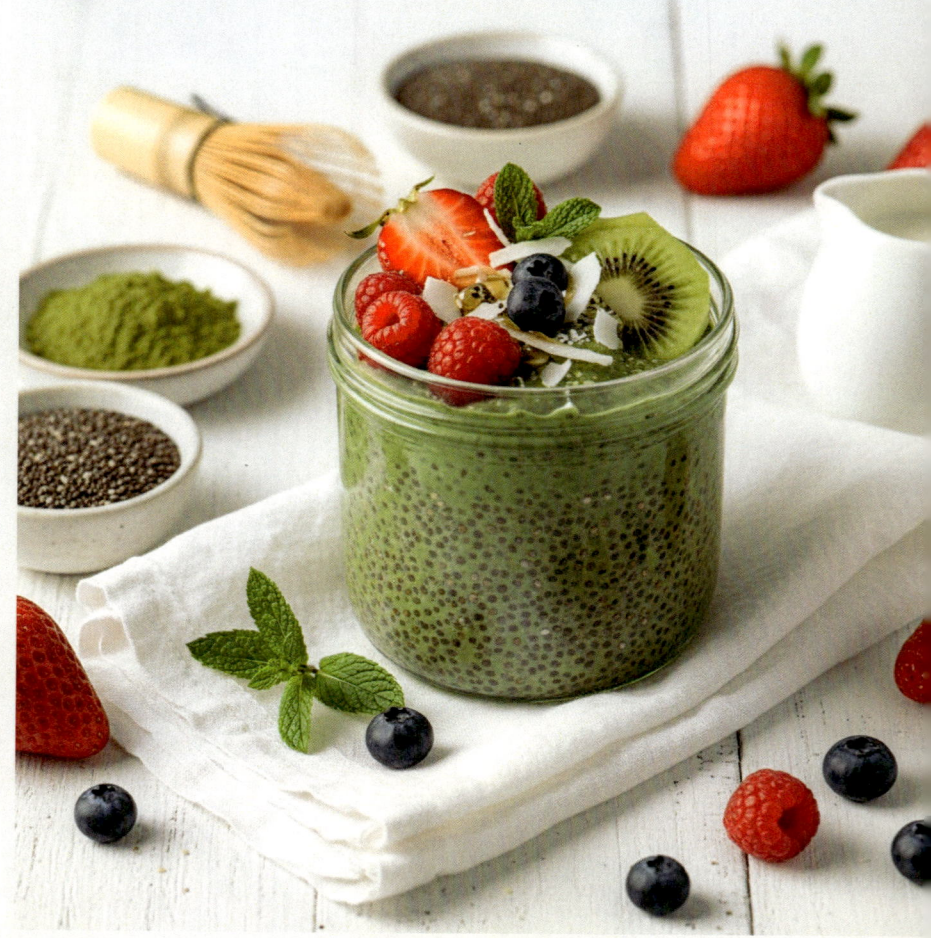

INSTRUCTIONS:

- Whisk almond milk, matcha, vanilla, maple syrup.
- Stir in chia seeds. Refrigerate overnight.
- Top with blueberries.

Sunshine Green Smoothie

Mantra: "I awaken my body with clarity."
Healing Note: Greens and pineapple provide hydration and energy.
Ancient Wisdom: Green foods have symbolized renewal and vitality across many traditions.

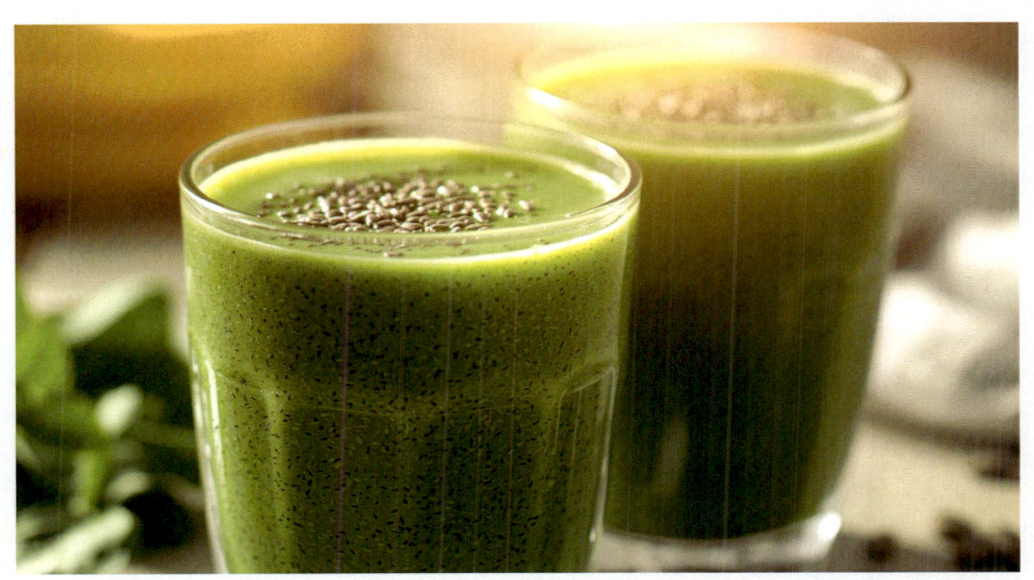

INGREDIENTS: (2 GLASSES)

- 2 cups spinach
- 1 banana
- 1 cup pineapple chunks
- 1 cup almond milk
- 1 tbsp chia seeds

INSTRUCTIONS:

- Blend all ingredients until smooth.
- Serve chilled.

Citrus Ginger Zinger Smoothie

Mantra: "I awaken my senses."
Healing Note: Citrus refreshes, ginger ignites energy.
Ancient Wisdom: Grapefruit was linked to cleansing in TCM.

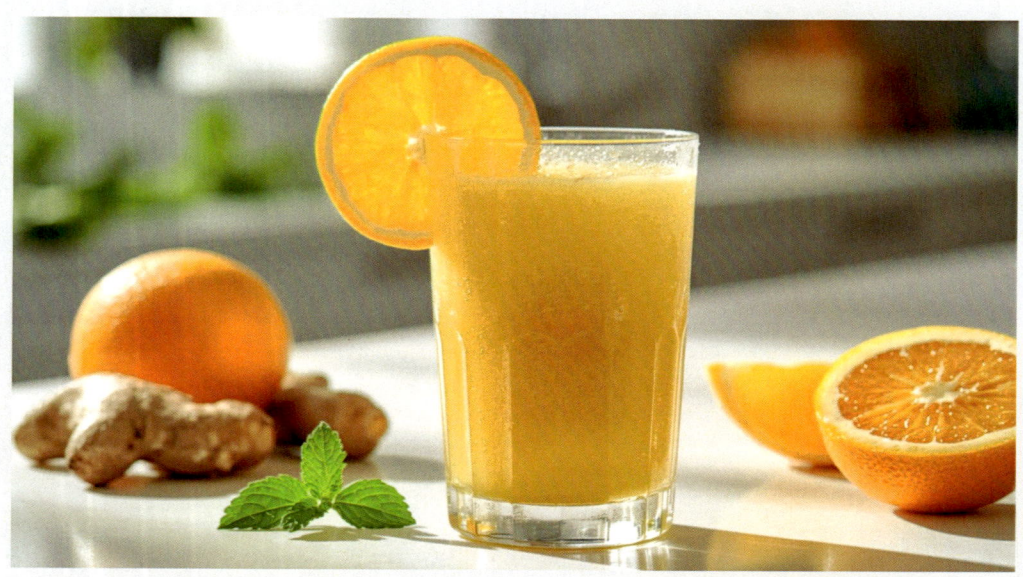

INGREDIENTS: (2 GLASSES)

- 1 orange, peeled
- ½ grapefruit, peeled
- 1 carrot, chopped
- 1 tsp fresh ginger
- 1 cup coconut water

INSTRUCTIONS:

- Blend all ingredients until smooth.
- Serve chilled.

Golden Turmeric Latte

Mantra: "I awaken my inner light and flow with radiant energy."

Healing Note: Turmeric supports joint health and reduces inflammation, while cinnamon and ginger enhance circulation and warmth. This latte awakens both body and intuition — a grounding yet energizing blend that balances your inner fire (agni) with calm focus.

Ancient Wisdom: Known in Ayurveda as Haldi Doodh, golden milk has been used for centuries as a healing tonic to restore energy, purify the body, and awaken spiritual radiance. Its golden color symbolizes the inner sun — a reminder of vitality, courage, and divine light within.

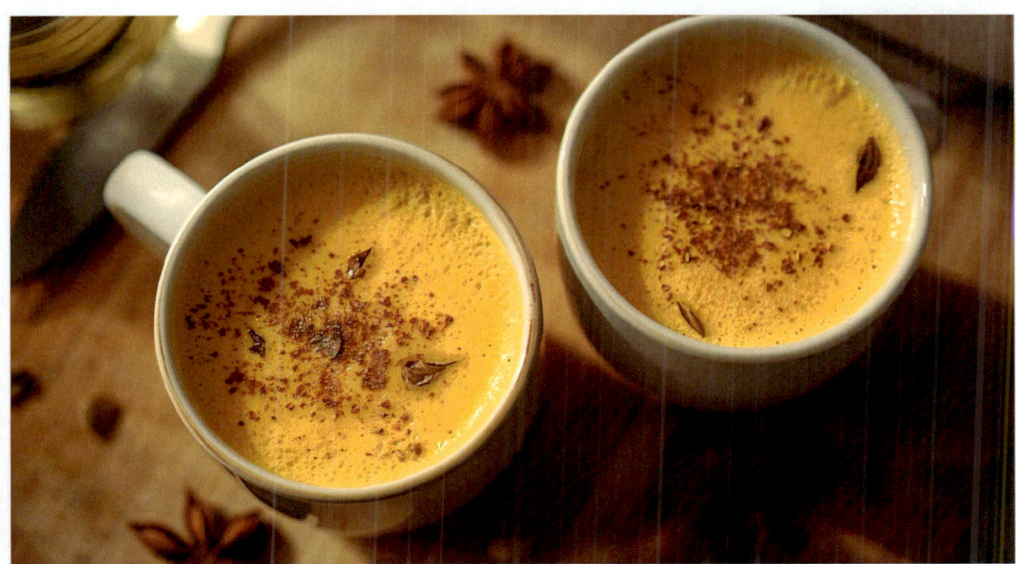

INGREDIENTS: (2 MUGS)

- 2 cups almond milk (or oat or coconut milk)
- 1 tsp ground turmeric
- ½ tsp cinnamon
- ¼ tsp ginger powder (or ½ tsp fresh grated ginger)
- Pinch of black pepper (enhances turmeric absorption)
- 1 tsp coconut oil (optional, for creaminess and absorption)
- 1 tsp honey or maple syrup (to taste)
- Sprinkle of cardamom or nutmeg (optional, for warmth and aroma)

INSTRUCTIONS:

- Warm milk gently in a small saucepan — do not boil.
- Whisk in turmeric, cinnamon, ginger, and black pepper until fully combined.
- Stir in coconut oil and sweetener; whisk until golden and frothy.
- Pour into mugs, sprinkle lightly with cardamom or nutmeg, and sip slowly.
- As you drink, breathe deeply — feel your body awakening and grounding in equal measure.

Citrus Turmeric Morning Tonic

Mantra: "I rise with radiant energy."
Healing Note: Turmeric reduces inflammation; citrus uplifts.
Ancient Wisdom: Citrus fruits were used in rituals to cleanse and energize.

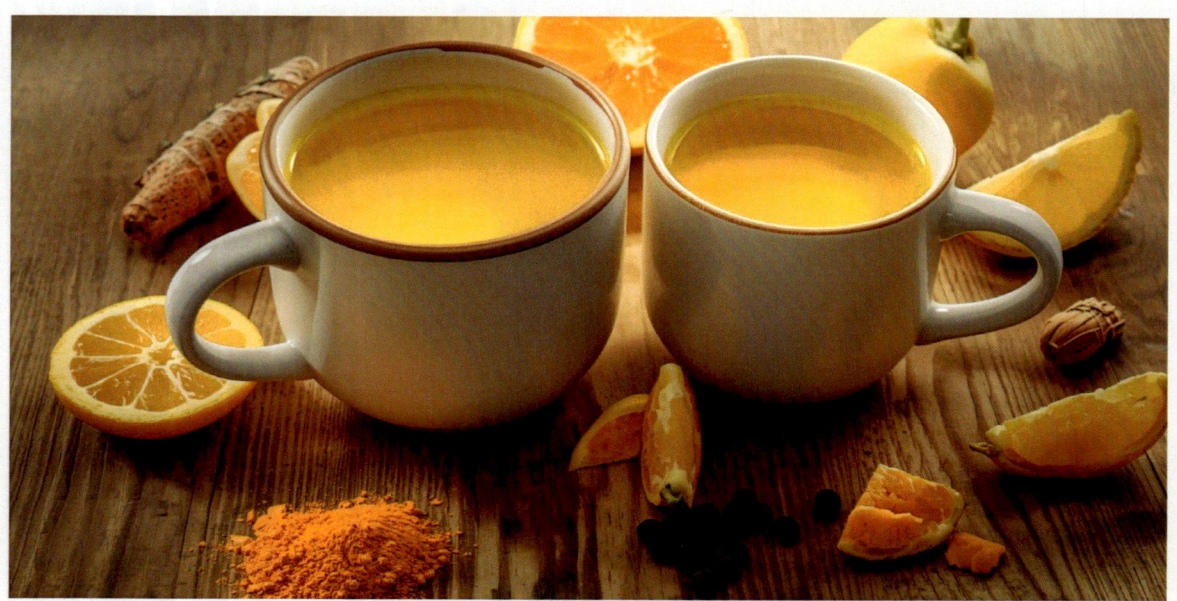

INGREDIENTS: (2 MUGS)

- Juice of 1 orange
- Juice of ½ lemon
- ½ tsp turmeric powder
- Pinch of black pepper
- 1 cup warm water

INSTRUCTIONS:

- Combine juices, turmeric, and pepper.
- Stir into warm water and sip slowly.

Lemon Chia Energy Bites

Mantra: "I embody fresh lightness."

Healing Note: Chia fuels steady energy.

Ancient Wisdom: Seeds have symbolized life-force energy for millennia.

INGREDIENTS: (12 BITES)

- 1 cup dates
- ½ cup cashews
- 2 tbsp chia seeds
- Zest of 1 lemon
- 1 tbsp coconut flakes

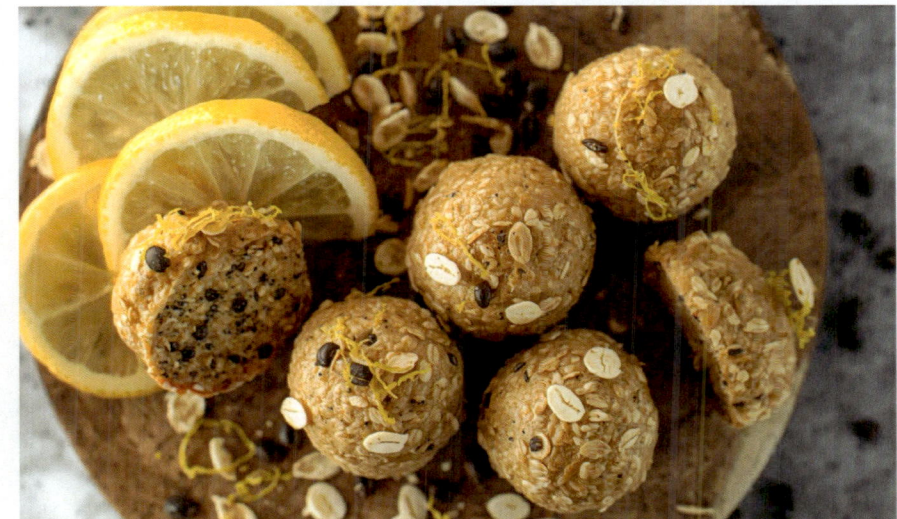

INSTRUCTIONS:

- Blend all ingredients in processor.
- Roll into balls.
- Chill 1 hour.

MANIFEST
Clarify Dreams & Align Actions

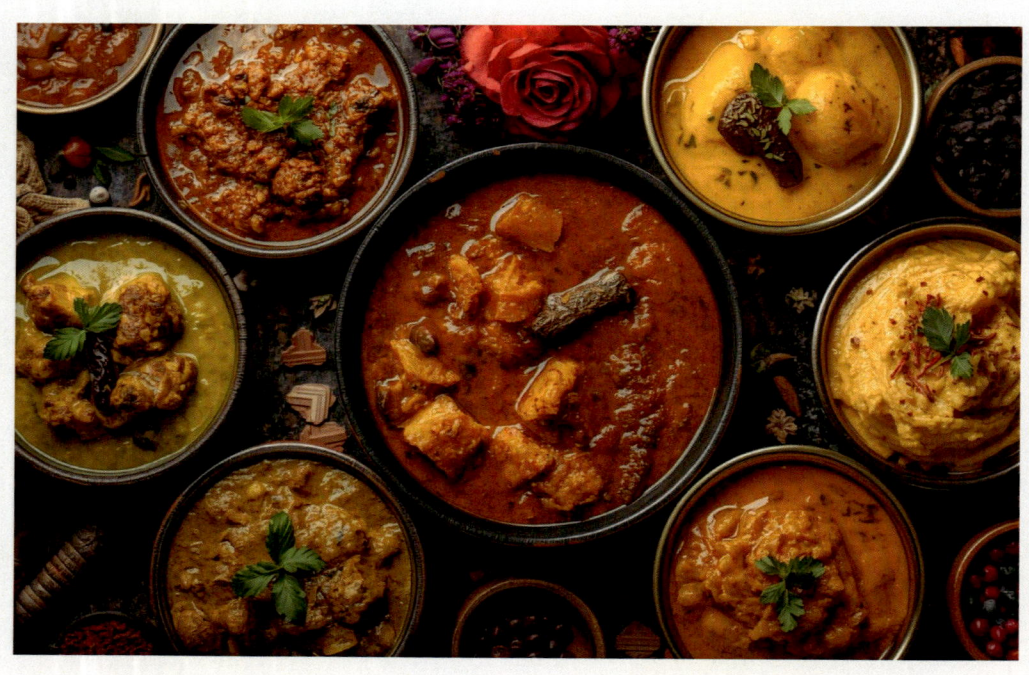

🍴 Optional Proteins & Cheeses

Manifest – Clarify Your Dreams

Mantra: "I align nourishment with my vision."
Healing Note: These proteins provide strength to bring ideas into form.
Ancient Wisdom: Lamb and cheese were central to Mediterranean feasts celebrating abundance and new beginnings.

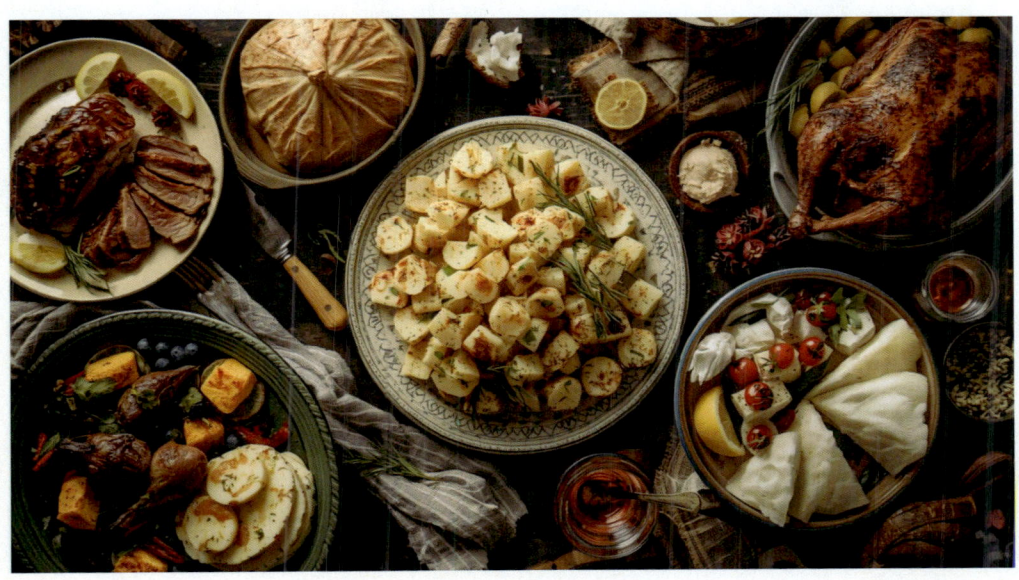

Meat (Lamb): Celebratory, rich in tradition.

Poultry (Duck/Chicken): Heartier, symbolic of abundance.

Seafood (Cod/Halibut): Clear, white fish for vision.

Cheese (Halloumi/Manchego): Firm, grounding, and versatile.

Dream Aligner Enchiladas

Mantra: "I align my actions with my vision."
Healing Note: Beans ground dreams into action.
Ancient Wisdom: Tortillas have fed generations as sacred daily bread.

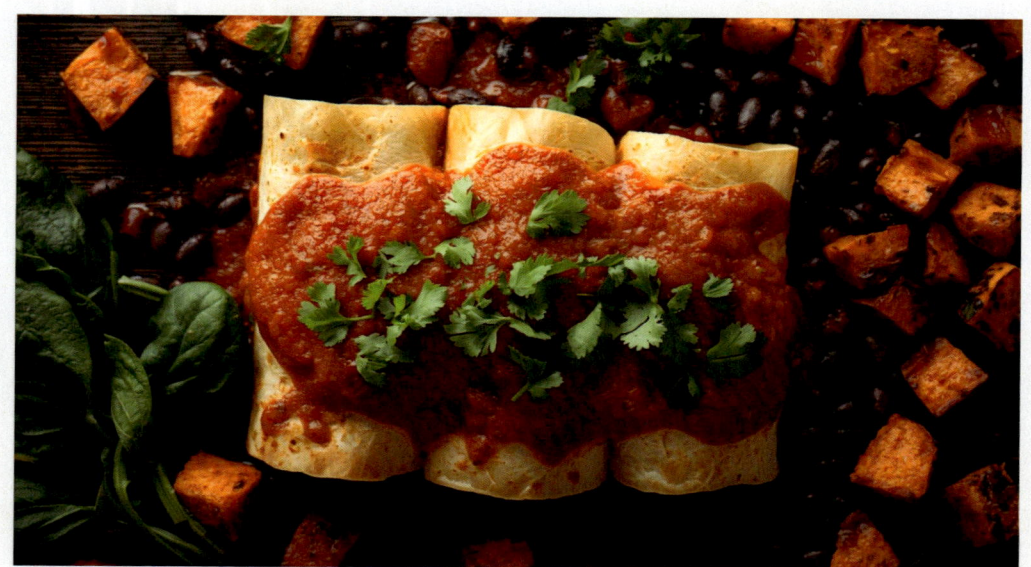

INGREDIENTS: (4 SERVINGS)

- 6 corn tortillas
- 1 cup black beans
- 1 cup sautéed spinach
- 1 cup roasted sweet potato
- Sauce: 1 cup tomato sauce + 1 tsp
  chili powder

INSTRUCTIONS:

- Fill tortillas with beans, spinach,
  sweet potato.
- Roll and place in baking dish.
- Cover with sauce; bake 20 minutes
  at 375°F.

Vision Aligner Mediterranean Chickpea Stew

Mantra: "I align with vision and clarity."

Healing Note: Chickpeas stabilize energy; Mediterranean spices ground while uplifting.

Ancient Wisdom: Stews were central to Mediterranean family tables, symbolizing shared dreams and communal abundance.

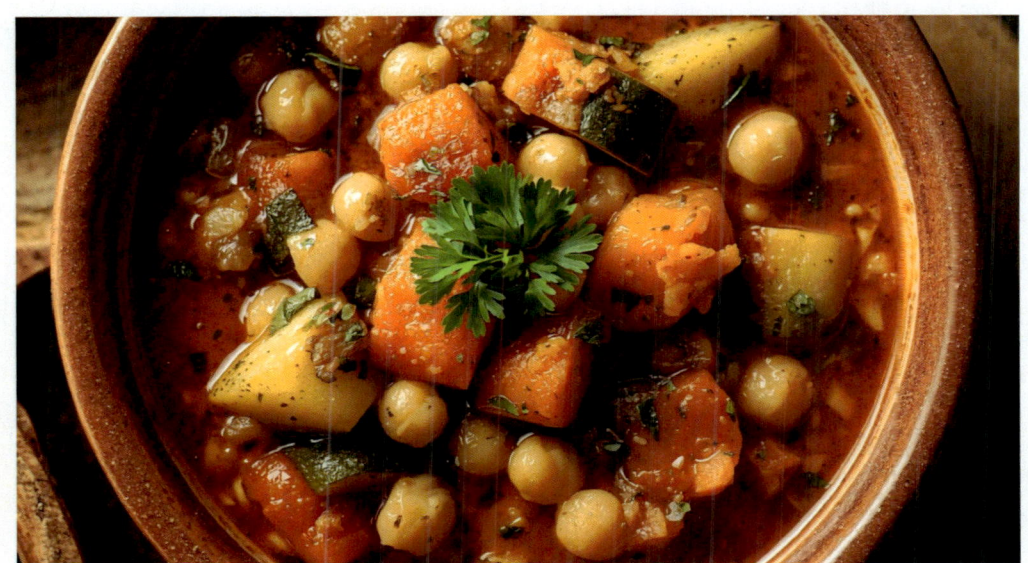

INGREDIENTS: (4 SERVINGS)

- 1 tbsp olive oil
- 1 onion, diced
- 2 garlic cloves, minced
- 2 carrots, chopped
- 1 zucchini, diced
- 1 can chickpeas, rinsed
- 1 can diced tomatoes
- 3 cups vegetable broth
- 1 tsp cumin
- 1 tsp smoked paprika
- 1 tsp oregano
- Salt & pepper
- Fresh parsley for garnish

INSTRUCTIONS:

- Heat olive oil in a pot. Sauté onion and garlic until fragrant.
- Add carrots and zucchini; cook 5 minutes.
- Stir in chickpeas, tomatoes, broth, and spices.
- Simmer 20–25 minutes until vegetables are tender.
- Garnish with fresh parsley and serve warm.

Dream Builder Stuffed Eggplant

Mantra: "I build my dreams with strength and vision."
Healing Note: Eggplant nourishes digestion; chickpeas sustain energy.
Ancient Wisdom: In Middle Eastern traditions, stuffed vegetables
symbolized abundance and hospitality.

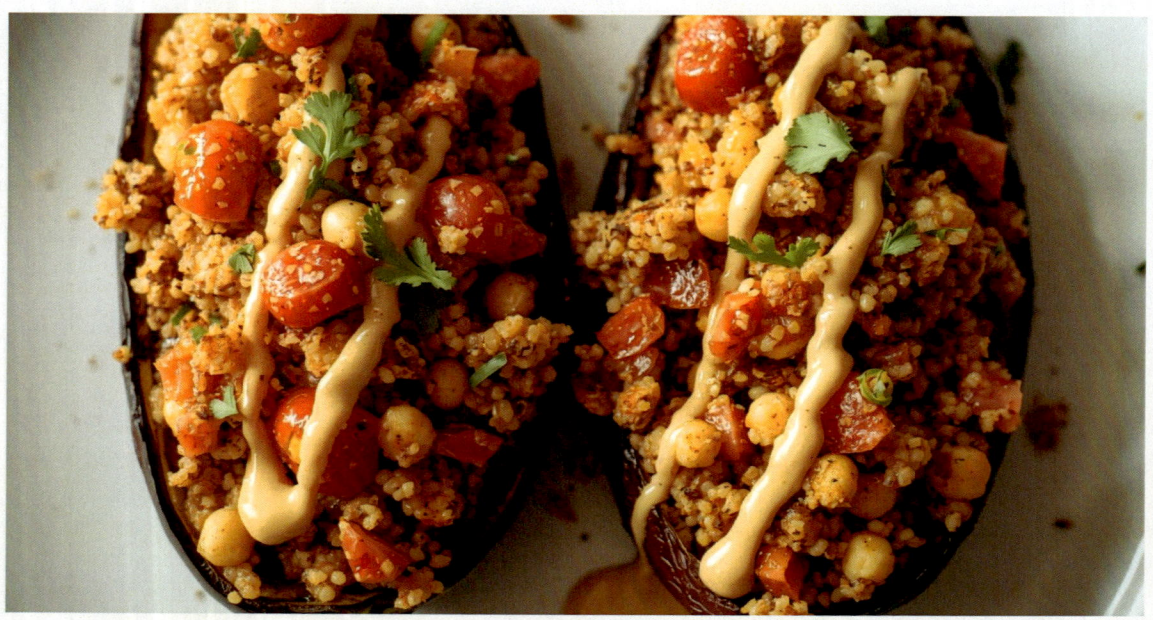

INGREDIENTS: (2 SERVINGS)

- 2 medium eggplants, halved lengthwise
- 1 tbsp olive oil
- 1 cup cooked quinoa
- 1 cup chickpeas
- 1 cup diced tomatoes
- 1 tsp cumin
- 1 tsp smoked paprika
- 2 tbsp tahini drizzle

INSTRUCTIONS:

- Scoop out eggplant flesh, brush shells with olive oil, and roast at 400°F for 20 minutes.
- Dice the scooped flesh and sauté with tomatoes, chickpeas, quinoa, cumin, and paprika.
- Stuff mixture into roasted shells.
- Drizzle with tahini and serve hot.

Rainbow Veggie Stir Fry

Mantra: "I bring color and creativity into my life."
Healing Note: Bright vegetables balance energy and uplift mood.
Ancient Wisdom: In Chinese traditions, eating a rainbow of vegetables symbolized balance of the five elements.

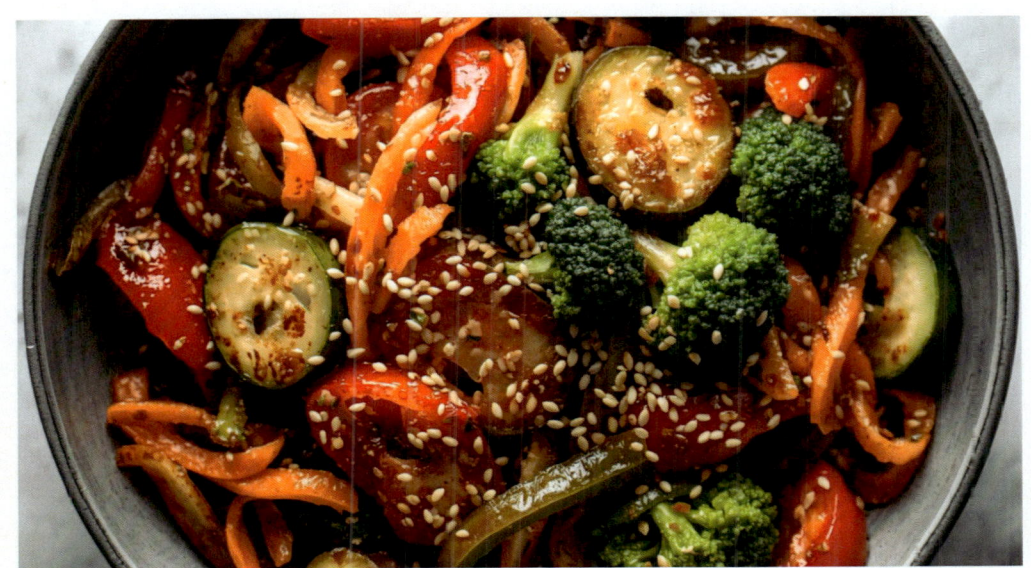

INGREDIENTS: (2 SERVINGS)

- 1 tbsp sesame oil
- 1 red bell pepper, sliced
- 1 zucchini, sliced
- 1 carrot, julienned
- 1 cup broccoli florets
- 2 tbsp tamari or soy sauce
- 1 tsp sesame seeds

INSTRUCTIONS:

- Heat oil; stir fry vegetables until tender-crisp.
- Add tamari; toss.
- Sprinkle sesame seeds before serving.

Black Bean Quinoa Bowl

Mantra: "I align with nourishment and vision."
Healing Note: Black beans provide grounding protein; quinoa uplifts with clarity.
Ancient Wisdom: Beans and corn were sacred "life foods" in Mesoamerican cultures, symbolizing harmony and sustenance.

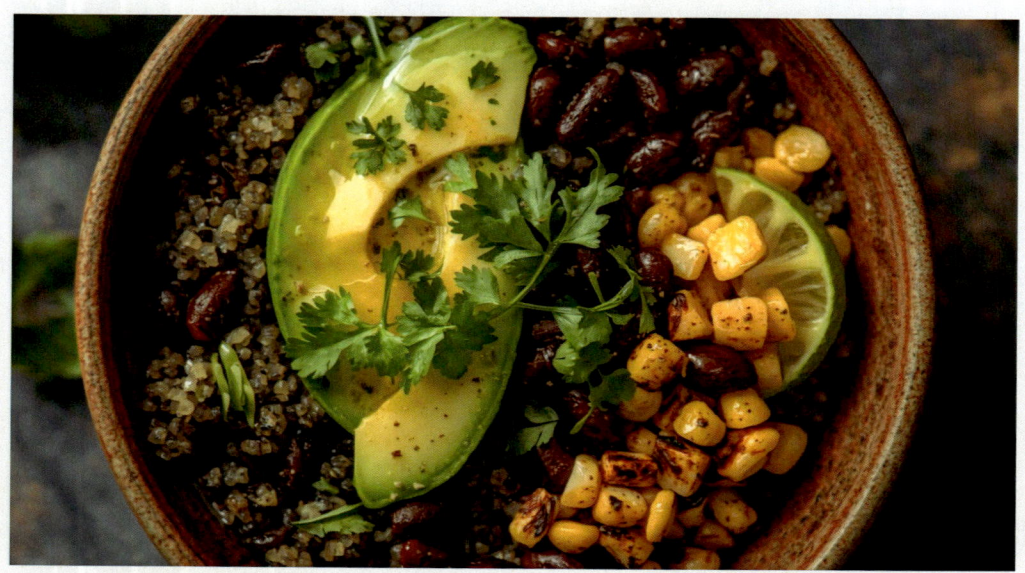

INGREDIENTS: (2 SERVINGS)

- 1 cup cooked quinoa
- 1 cup black beans
- ½ avocado, sliced
- 1 cup roasted corn
- 1 tbsp olive oil + juice of 1 lime
- Fresh cilantro

INSTRUCTIONS:

- Layer quinoa, beans, corn, and avocado in bowls.
- Drizzle with olive oil and lime juice.
- Garnish with cilantro.

Dream Aligner Pesto Pasta with Spinach & Sun-Dried Tomatoes

Mantra: "I align thought, heart, and action with purpose."

Healing Note: Spinach nourishes the heart and blood, while walnuts strengthen the brain and nervous system — promoting focus and flow for turning dreams into reality.

Ancient Wisdom: Pesto originated as a sacred "green paste" of renewal and prosperity in early Mediterranean rituals, symbolizing fresh beginnings and creative energy.

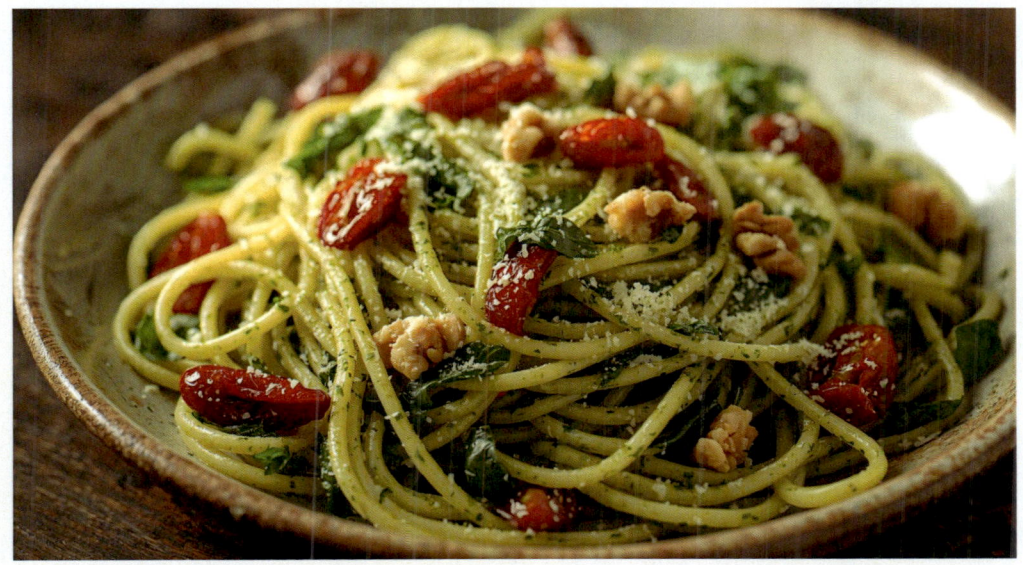

INGREDIENTS: (2 SERVINGS)

- 6 oz spaghetti or linguine (gluten-free if desired)
- 2 cups baby spinach
- ¼ cup sun-dried tomatoes, chopped
- ¼ cup walnuts or pine nuts
- 1 garlic clove
- 2 tbsp olive oil
- Juice of ½ lemon
- Salt & pepper to taste
- Optional: 2 tbsp nutritional yeast or Parmesan for richness

INSTRUCTIONS:

- Cook pasta according to package directions.
- Blend spinach, walnuts, garlic, olive oil, lemon, and seasoning into a smooth pesto.
- Toss pasta with pesto and sun-dried tomatoes.
- Sprinkle with nutritional yeast or Parmesan and serve warm.

Dreamer's Mango Avocado Salad

Mantra: "I embody joy and possibility."
Healing Note: Mango uplifts mood; avocado nourishes heart energy.
Ancient Wisdom: In Ayurveda, mango was considered a fruit of the gods, symbolizing prosperity.

INGREDIENTS: (2 SERVINGS)

- 2 cups baby spinach
- 1 ripe mango, diced
- 1 avocado, diced
- ¼ cup red onion, thinly sliced
- 2 tbsp pumpkin seeds
- Dressing: juice of 1 lime, 2 tbsp olive oil, pinch sea salt

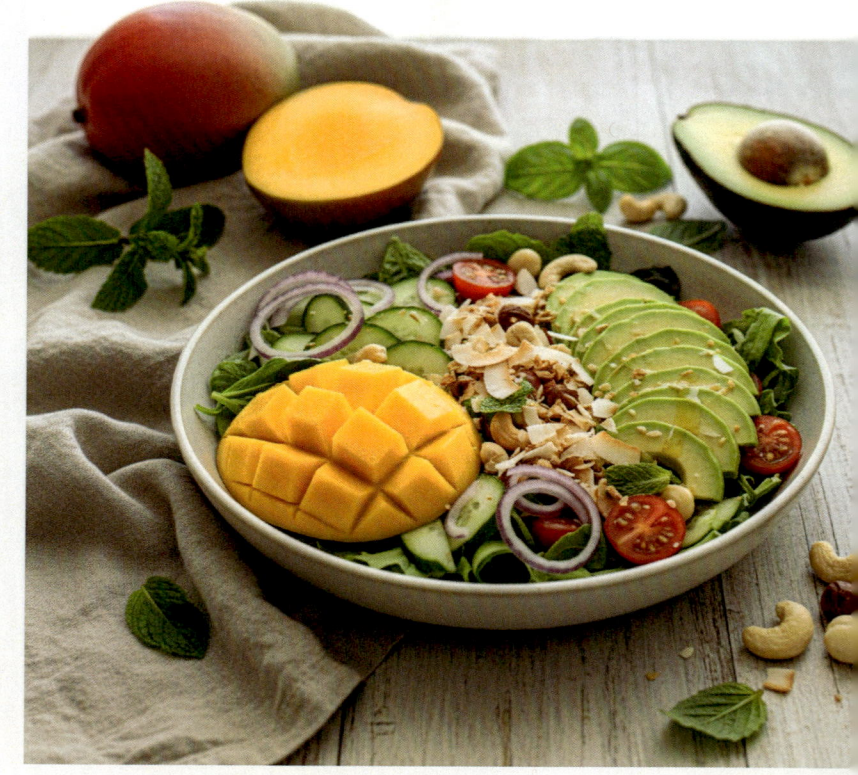

INSTRUCTIONS:

- Layer spinach, mango, avocado, onion in a bowl.
- Whisk lime juice, olive oil, salt. Drizzle over salad.
- Sprinkle pumpkin seeds; toss gently.

Vision Noodle Stir Fry

Mantra: "I align with flow and creativity."
Healing Note: Rainbow veggies energize; sesame oil grounds clarity.
Ancient Wisdom: In Chinese culture, long noodles symbolize longevity and prosperous vision.

INGREDIENTS: (2 SERVINGS)

- 4 oz rice noodles, cooked
- 1 cup broccoli florets
- 1 red bell pepper, sliced
- 1 cup snap peas
- 1 carrot, julienned
- 2 tbsp tamari or soy sauce
- 1 tbsp sesame oil
- 1 tsp ginger, grated
- 1 clove garlic, minced
- Sesame seeds for garnish

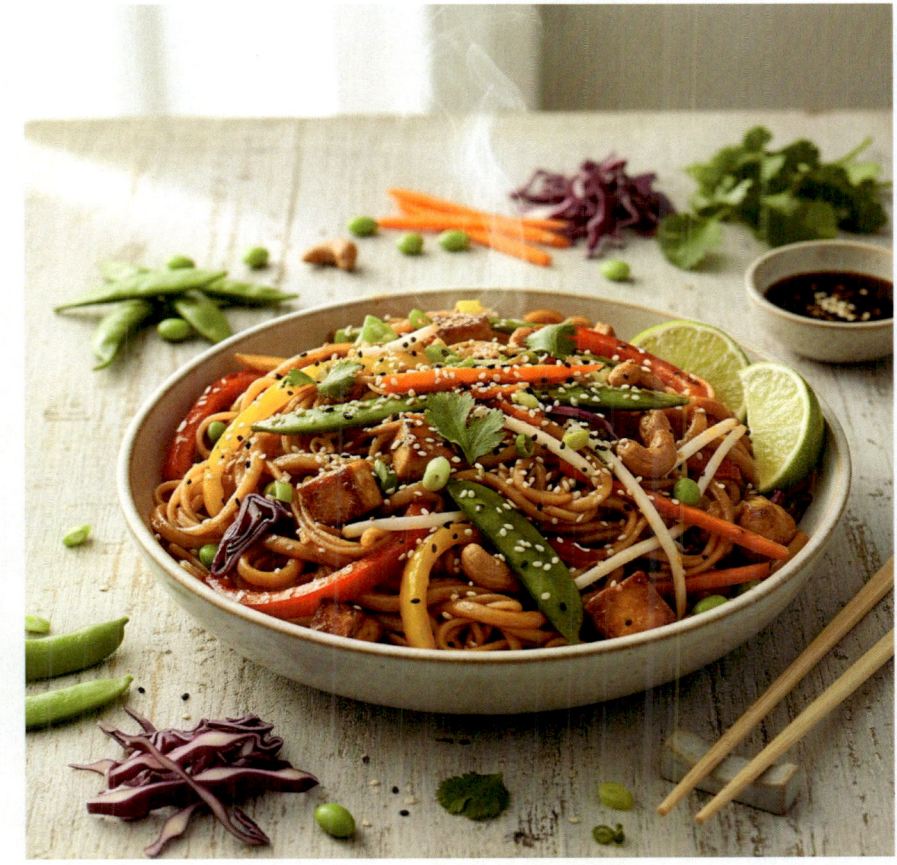

INSTRUCTIONS:

- Cook noodles per package; drain.
- Stir fry veggies in sesame oil with garlic + ginger 5 minutes.
- Add noodles + tamari, toss well.
- Sprinkle sesame seeds to serve.

Radiance Black Bean Tacos

Mantra: "I act on my vision with courage."
Healing Note: Black beans sustain energy; sweet potato grounds manifestation into reality.
Ancient Wisdom: Beans were revered in Mesoamerica as sacred life-giving foods.

INGREDIENTS: (2 SERVINGS – 4 TACOS)

- 4 corn tortillas
- 1 cup black beans, rinsed
- 1 cup roasted sweet potato cubes
- 1 cup shredded red cabbage
- ½ avocado, sliced
- Lime wedges
- Optional toppings:
- Fresh salsa or pico de gallo
- Chopped cilantro
- Crumbled feta or vegan cheese
- Toasted pumpkin seeds for crunch

INSTRUCTIONS:

- Prepare the filling: Heat olive oil in a skillet. Add garlic, cumin, paprika, and chili powder; stir 30 seconds until fragrant.
- Add black beans and mash lightly with a fork, leaving some texture. Cook 3–5 minutes until warm and seasoned.
- Stir in roasted sweet potato cubes if using. Add salt, pepper, and lime juice to taste.
- Assemble tacos: Warm tortillas. Spoon the black bean mixture into each.
- Top with cabbage, avocado, and any optional garnishes. Serve immediately with extra lime wedges.

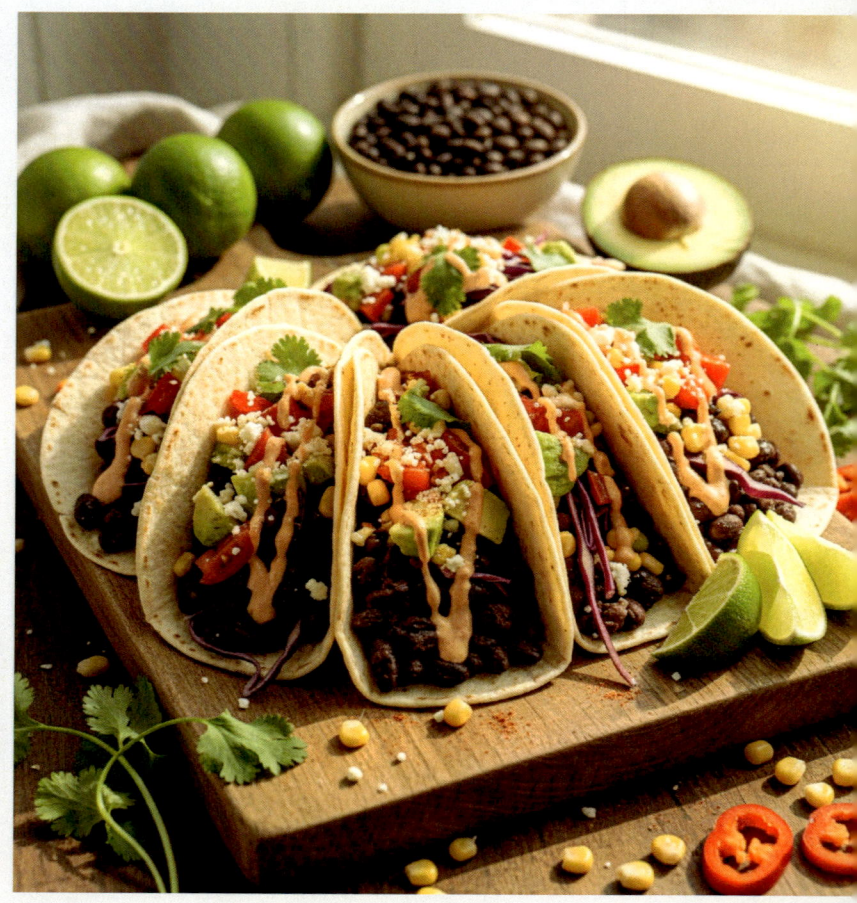

Chickpea Curry

Mantra: "I nourish courage and clarity."

Healing Note: Chickpeas give steady energy; curry spices boost circulation and warmth.

Ancient Wisdom: In Ayurveda, curry spices like turmeric and cumin were blended for balance, resilience, and digestive fire (agni).

INGREDIENTS: (4 SERVINGS)

- 1 tbsp coconut or olive oil
- 1 onion, diced
- 2 cloves garlic, minced
- 1 tbsp curry powder (or 2 tsp garam masala + 1 tsp turmeric)
- 1 can (14 oz) coconut milk
- 1 can (15 oz) chickpeas, rinsed and drained
- 1 cup vegetable broth or water
- 2 cups baby spinach
- 1 cup diced tomatoes (optional)
- ½–1 tsp salt & pepper
- Juice of ½ lime
- Fresh cilantro for garnish (optional)

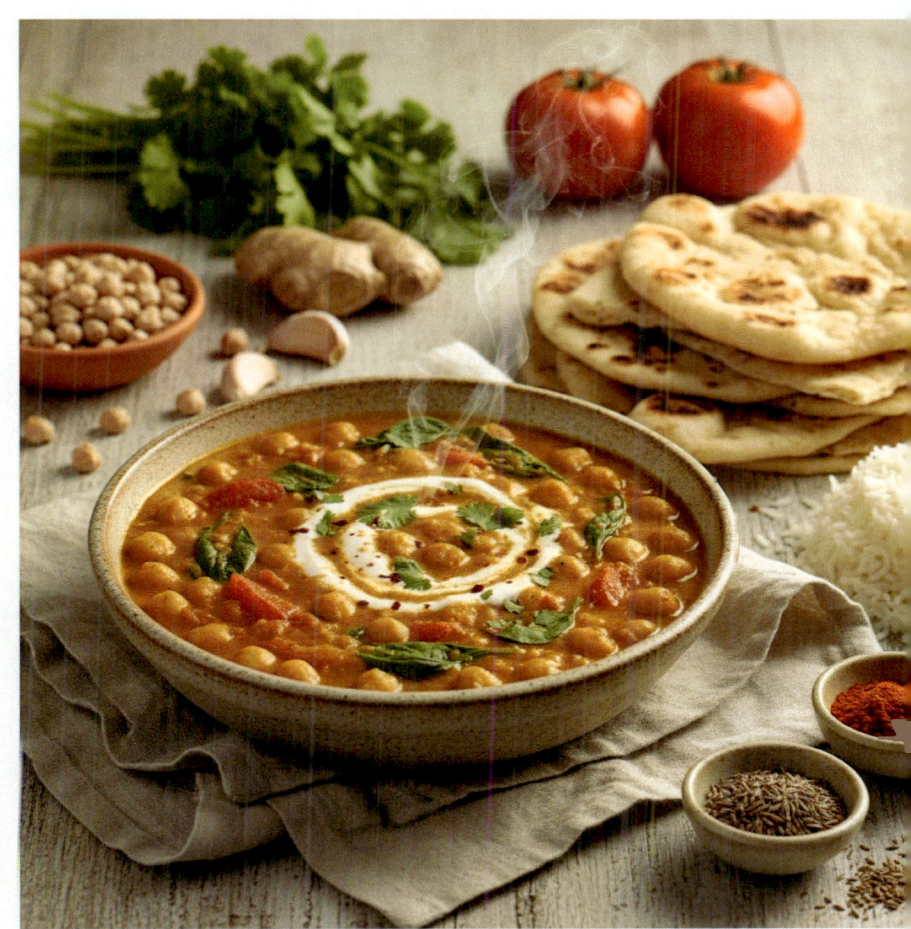

INSTRUCTIONS:

- Heat oil in a large pot. Sauté onion 4 minutes; add garlic 1 minute.
- Stir in curry powder; toast 30 seconds to release aroma.
- Add coconut milk, broth, chickpeas (and tomatoes if using). Simmer 12–15 minutes.
- Stir in spinach until just wilted.
- Season with salt, pepper, and lime juice. Garnish with cilantro.

Strawberry Rose Elixir

Mantra: "I attract beauty and possibility."
Healing Note: Strawberries open the heart; rose soothes emotions.
Ancient Wisdom: Rose water has been used in Persian ceremonies for love.

INGREDIENTS: (2 SERVINGS)

- 1 cup strawberries
- 1 cup almond milk
- 1 tsp rose water
- 1 tsp honey (optional)

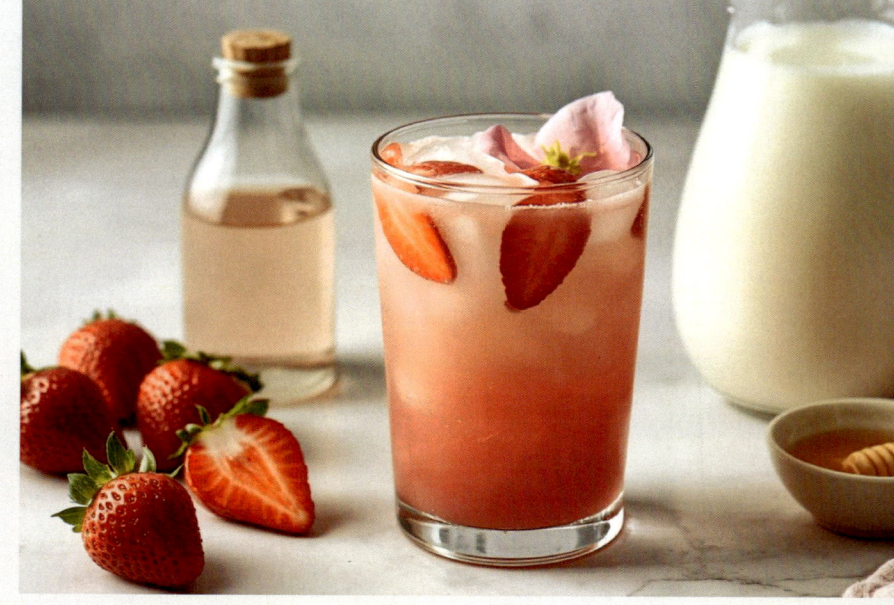

INSTRUCTIONS:

- Blend all ingredients until smooth.
- Serve chilled.

Abundance Glow Smoothie

Mantra: "I glow with clarity and joy."
Healing Note: Fruits provide natural energy and antioxidants.
Ancient Wisdom: Strawberries were linked to love and fertility in ancient Roman traditions.

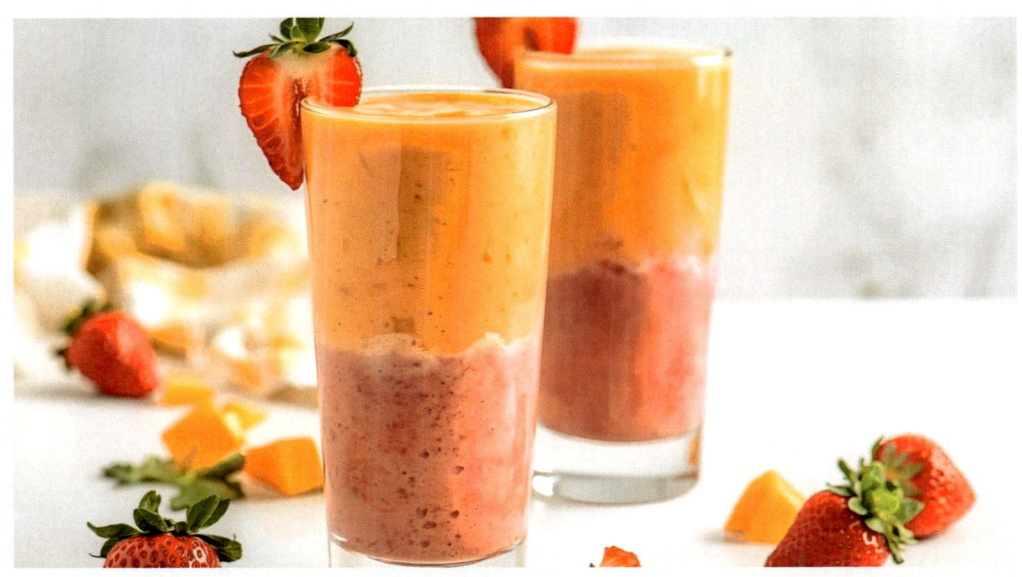

INGREDIENTS: (2 GLASSES)

- 1 cup strawberries
- 1 cup mango
- 1 banana
- 1 cup almond milk
- 1 tsp flaxseeds

INSTRUCTIONS:

- Blend all ingredients until smooth.
- Serve chilled.

Cacao Power Latte

Mantra: "I align my actions with my dreams."
Healing Note: Cacao uplifts mood and opens the heart; cinnamon steadies blood sugar and energy.
Ancient Wisdom: The Mayans and Aztecs drank cacao in ceremonies, believing it connected them to spirit and courage.

INGREDIENTS: (2 MUGS)

- 2 cups unsweetened almond or oat milk
- 2 tbsp raw cacao powder (or unsweetened cocoa)
- 1 tsp cinnamon
- 1–2 tsp maple syrup or honey (optional)
- Pinch sea salt
- Pinch cayenne or ginger powder (optional, for extra warmth)

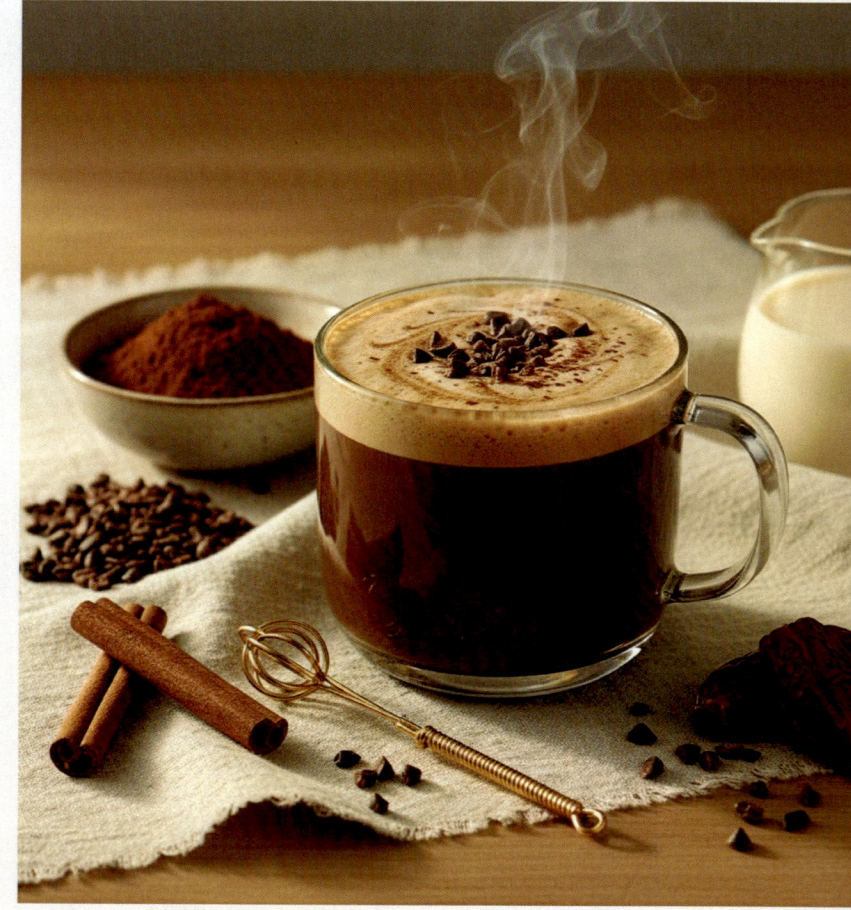

INSTRUCTIONS:

- Warm milk in a small pot over medium heat.
- Whisk in cacao, cinnamon, maple/honey, salt, and optional cayenne or ginger.
- Froth with a whisk or blender if desired.
- Pour into mugs, sip slowly with intention.

Cacao Almond Dream Bars

Mantra: "I savor sweet abundance."
Healing Note: Cacao uplifts; almonds strengthen clarity.
Ancient Wisdom: Cacao rituals connected spirit and abundance.

INGREDIENTS: (12 BARS)

- Base: 1 cup oats + ½ cup almonds + 6 dates
- Filling: ¼ cup cacao + 2 tbsp almond butter + 2 tbsp maple
- Topping: coconut flakes

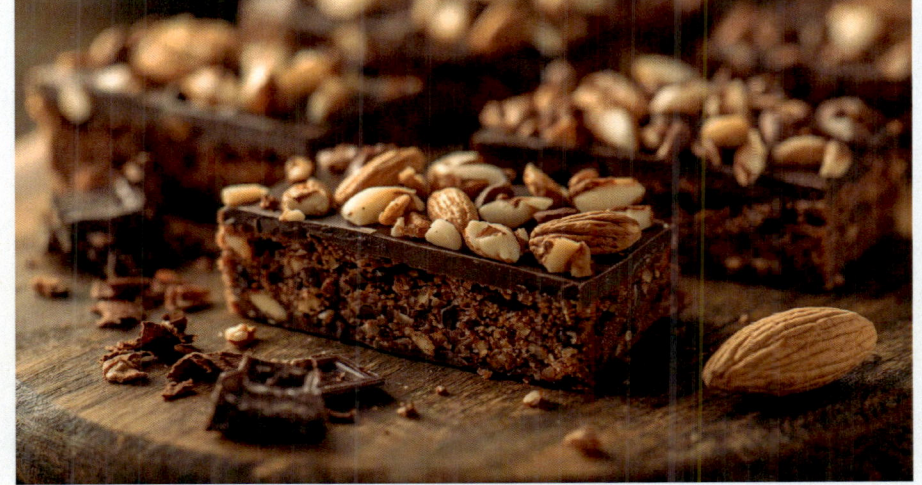

INSTRUCTIONS:

- Blend base, press into pan.
- Mix filling, spread on top.
- Sprinkle coconut; refrigerate 2 hrs.

Almond Bliss Balls

Mantra: "I embody sweetness, strength, and ease."

Healing Note: Almonds provide protein and healthy fats that stabilize energy and soothe the nervous system. Dates offer natural sweetness that balances blood sugar while uplifting mood — a perfect snack for sustaining energy with joy and intention.

Ancient Wisdom: In ancient Persian and Indian traditions, almonds symbolized prosperity, vitality, and divine favor. Sharing almond sweets was seen as a gesture of love, abundance, and well-being — nourishment for both body and soul.

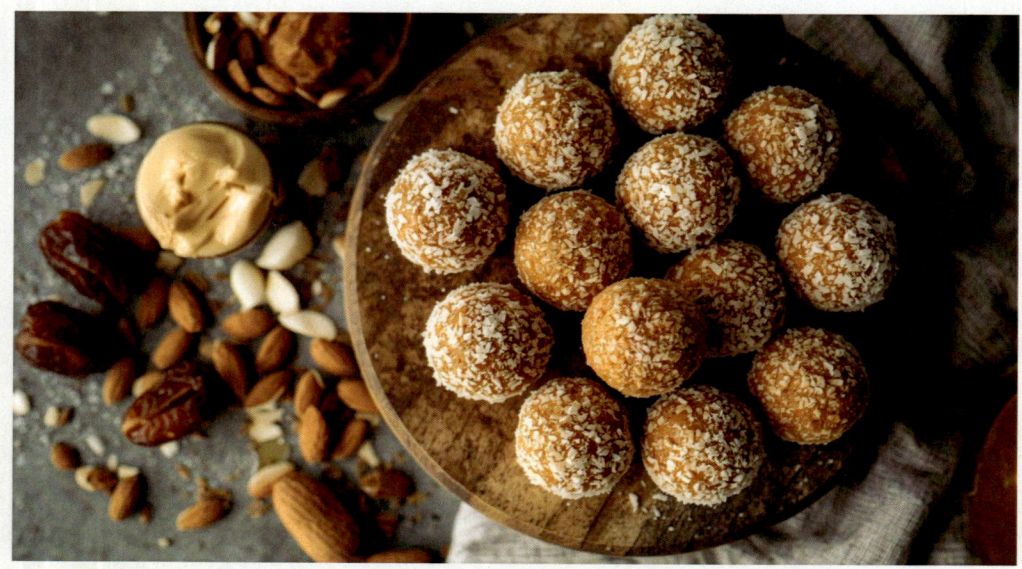

INGREDIENTS: (12 BALLS)

- 1 cup raw almonds
- 6 Medjool dates, pitted
- 2 tbsp almond butter
- 1 tbsp honey or maple syrup
- 2 tbsp shredded coconut (plus extra for rolling)
- 1 tsp vanilla extract
- Pinch of sea salt
- Optional Add-ins:
- 1 tsp cacao powder (for chocolate version)
- 1 tbsp chia seeds (for extra energy boost)

INSTRUCTIONS:

- Add almonds to a food processor and pulse until finely ground.
- Add dates, almond butter, honey or maple syrup, coconut, vanilla, and salt.
- Process until mixture sticks together (add 1 tsp water if too dry).
- Roll into 1-inch balls using your hands.
- Coat each ball in shredded coconut for texture and beauty.
- Chill in refrigerator for at least 30 minutes before serving.

PILLAR 4
EVOLVE
RELEASE & EMBRACE GROWTH

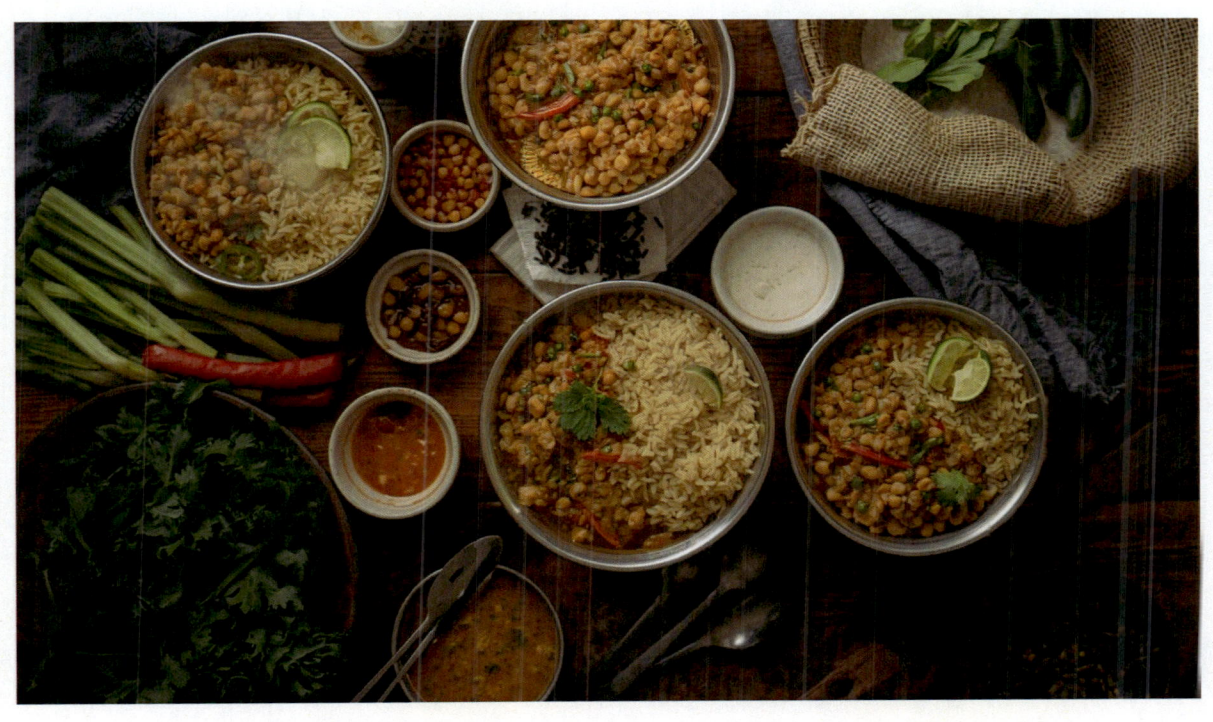

¶¶ Optional Proteins & Cheeses

Evolve – Release & Embrace Growth

Mantra: "I release heaviness and grow with ease."
Healing Note: Light proteins support renewal and digestion.
Ancient Wisdom: Water-based foods like fish were seen as guides of change and adaptability

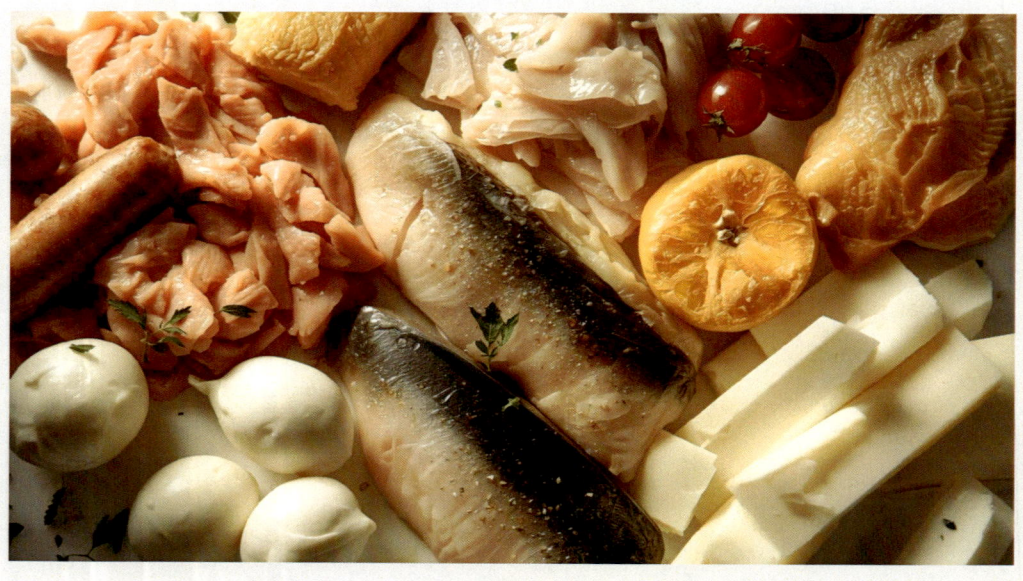

Meat (Turkey/Chicken Sausage): Lighter protein.
Poultry (Poached Chicken): Gentle, easy to digest.
Seafood (Trout/Tilapia): Flaky and flowing.
Cheese (Fresh Mozzarella): Mild, simple, cleansing.

Lentil Detox Soup

Mantra: "I release with ease."
Healer's Note: Lentils + greens support detox and renewal.
Ancient Wisdom: Lentils were sacred foods of purification across cultures.

INGREDIENTS: (4 SERVINGS)

- 1 tbsp olive oil
- 1 onion, diced
- 2 carrots, chopped
- 2 celery stalks, chopped
- 2 cloves garlic, minced
- 1 cup green lentils
- 6 cups veggie broth
- 2 cups kale or spinach, chopped
- 1 tsp cumin
- ½ tsp turmeric
- Salt + pepper

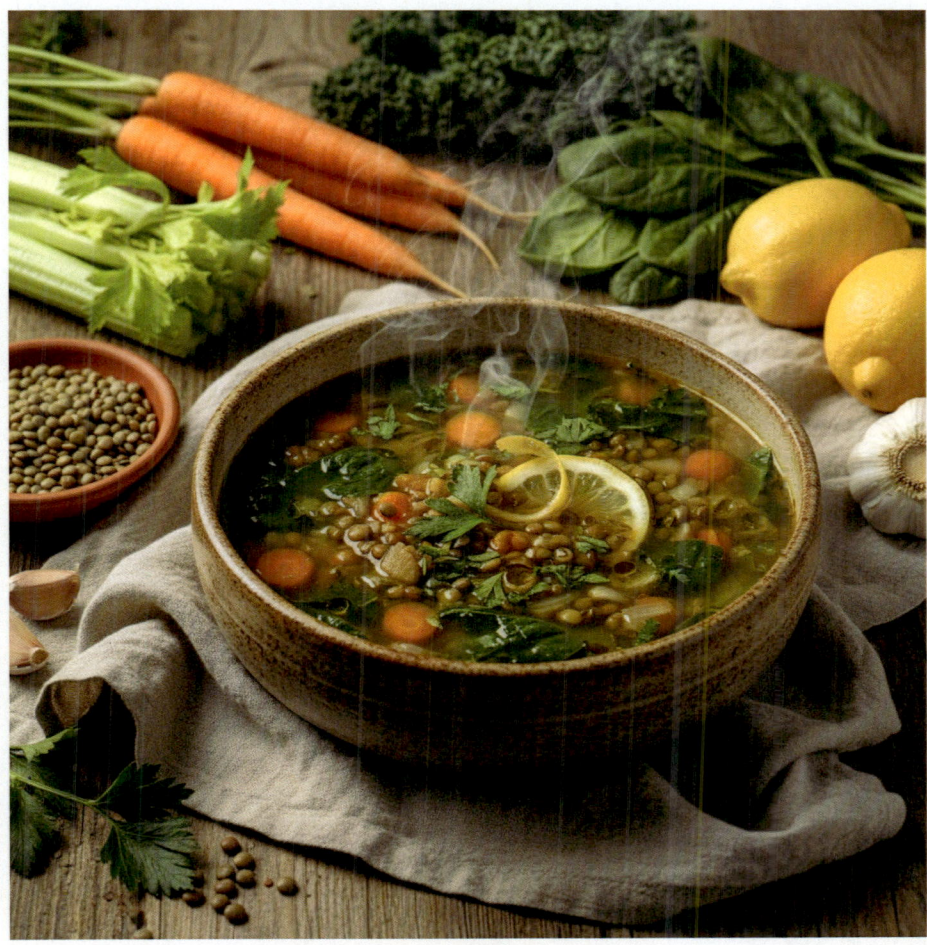

INSTRUCTIONS:

- Sauté onion, garlic, carrots, celery. Add lentils, broth, spices. Simmer 30 min. Stir in greens before serving.

Spaghetti Squash Glow Bowl

Mantra: "I transform with grace and ease."
Healing Note: Spaghetti squash is low-carb, hydrating, and rich in fiber for gentle renewal.
Ancient Wisdom: Squash was a staple in Indigenous "Three Sisters" gardens, symbolizing nourishment, protection, and cycles of growth.

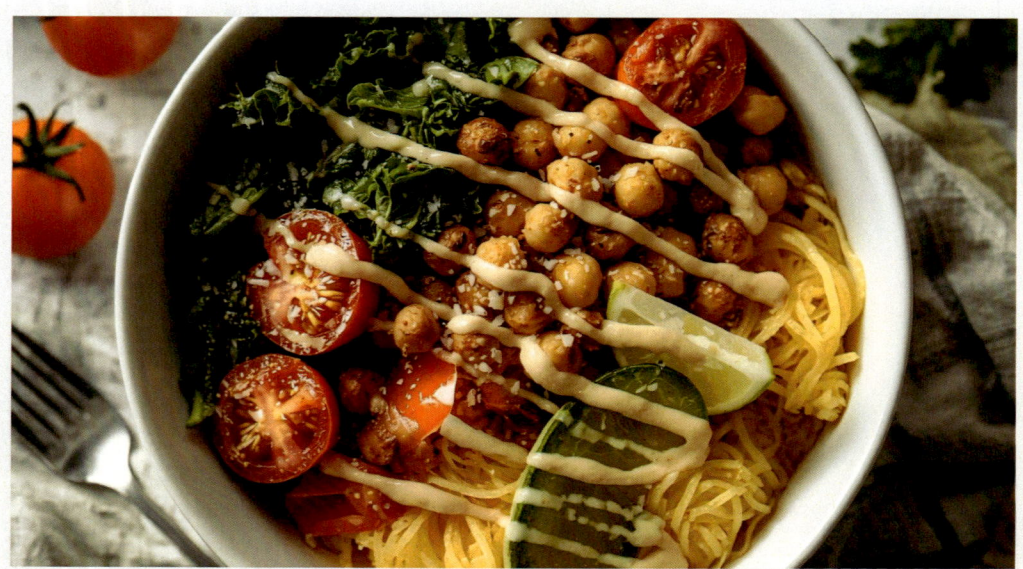

INGREDIENTS: (2-3 SERVINGS)

- 1 medium spaghetti squash
- 1 tbsp olive oil
- 2 cups spinach or kale, lightly sautéed
- 1 cup cherry tomatoes, halved
- ½ cup chickpeas, roasted or pan-fried
- 2 tbsp tahini
- Juice of ½ lemon
- Pinch of salt & pepper

INSTRUCTIONS:

- Preheat oven to 400°F. Cut squash in half, remove seeds, drizzle with olive oil. Roast face-down for 40 minutes until tender.
- Scrape the flesh with a fork to form "noodles."
- Top with greens, cherry tomatoes, and chickpeas.
- Whisk tahini, lemon juice, salt & pepper; drizzle over bowl.

Renewal Veggie & Tempeh Stir-Fry

Mantra: "I grow stronger as I release what no longer serves me."
Healing Note: Tempeh provides clean protein; ginger aids release and renewal.
Ancient Wisdom: Fermented foods like tempeh have symbolized transformation and longevity in Asian traditions.

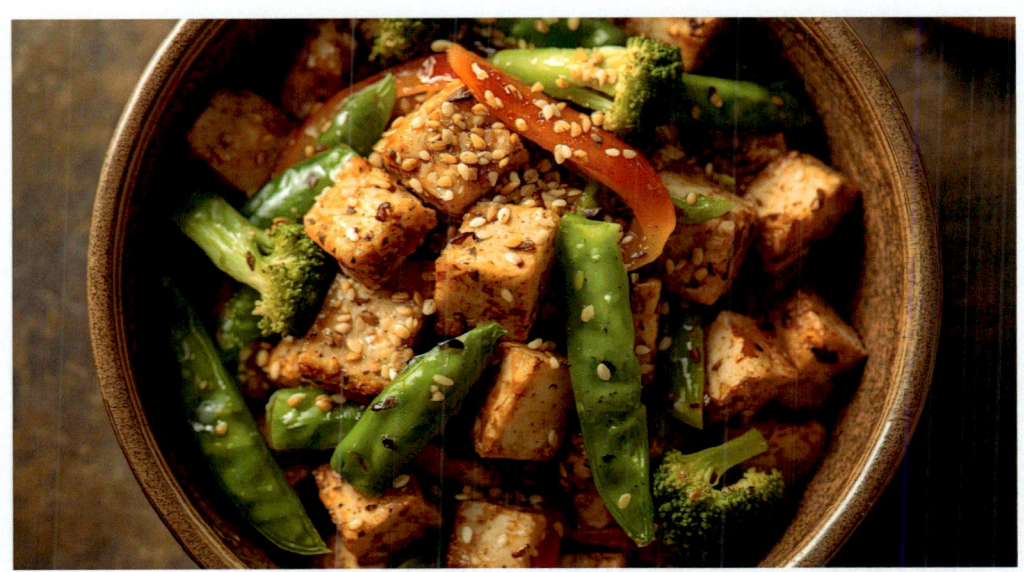

INGREDIENTS: (2 SERVINGS)

- 1 tbsp sesame oil
- 1 block tempeh, cubed
- 1 cup broccoli florets
- 1 cup snap peas
- 1 red bell pepper, sliced
- 2 tbsp tamari or soy sauce
- 1 tbsp grated ginger
- 1 tsp sesame seeds

INSTRUCTIONS:

- Heat sesame oil in wok; sauté tempeh until golden.
- Add broccoli, peas, and bell pepper; cook 5 minutes.
- Add tamari and ginger; stir fry 2 more minutes.
- Sprinkle sesame seeds before serving.

Light Mung Bean & Vegetable Curry

Mantra: "I flow with change and embrace transformation."
Healing Note: Mung beans are detoxifying and protein-rich; turmeric and lime balance digestion and refresh the body.
Ancient Wisdom: In Ayurveda, mung beans are considered tridoshic — balancing all energies for purification and renewal.

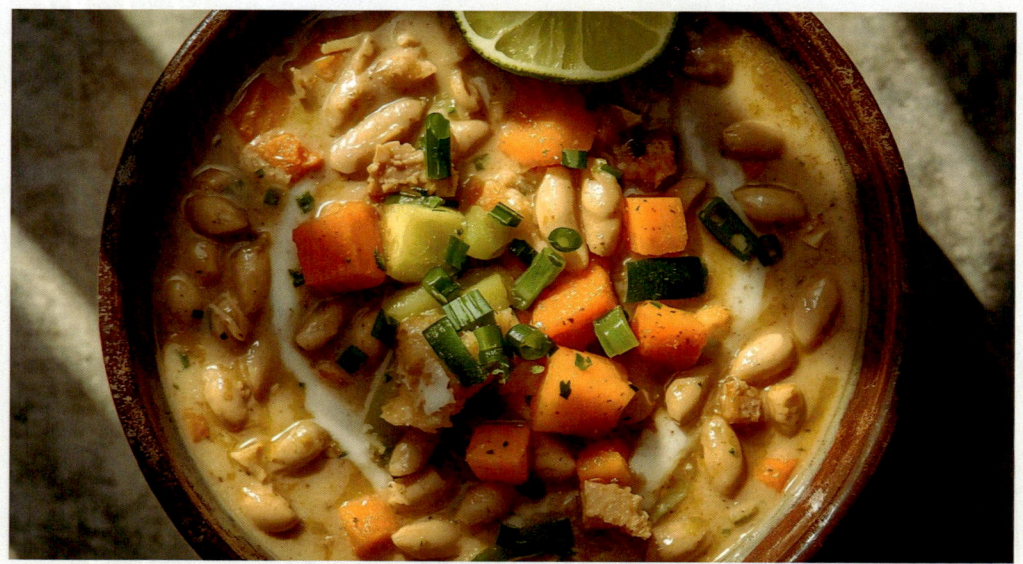

INGREDIENTS: (4 SERVINGS)

- 1 tbsp coconut oil
- 1 onion, chopped
- 2 garlic cloves, minced
- 1 tsp grated ginger
- 1 cup mung beans, soaked overnight
- 1 cup diced carrots
- 1 zucchini, chopped
- 1 tsp turmeric
- 1 tsp cumin
- 1 can coconut milk
- 2 cups vegetable broth
- Juice of ½ lime

INSTRUCTIONS:

- Sauté onion, garlic, and ginger in coconut oil until fragrant.
- Add turmeric, cumin, and mung beans; stir for 1 minute.
- Add carrots, zucchini, coconut milk, and broth.
- Simmer 25–30 minutes until beans are tender.
- Finish with lime juice.

Spring Renewal Stir Fry

Mantra: "I release the old and grow into the new."
Healing Note: Greens refresh; miso balances gut health.
Ancient Wisdom: Fermented foods symbolize transformation.

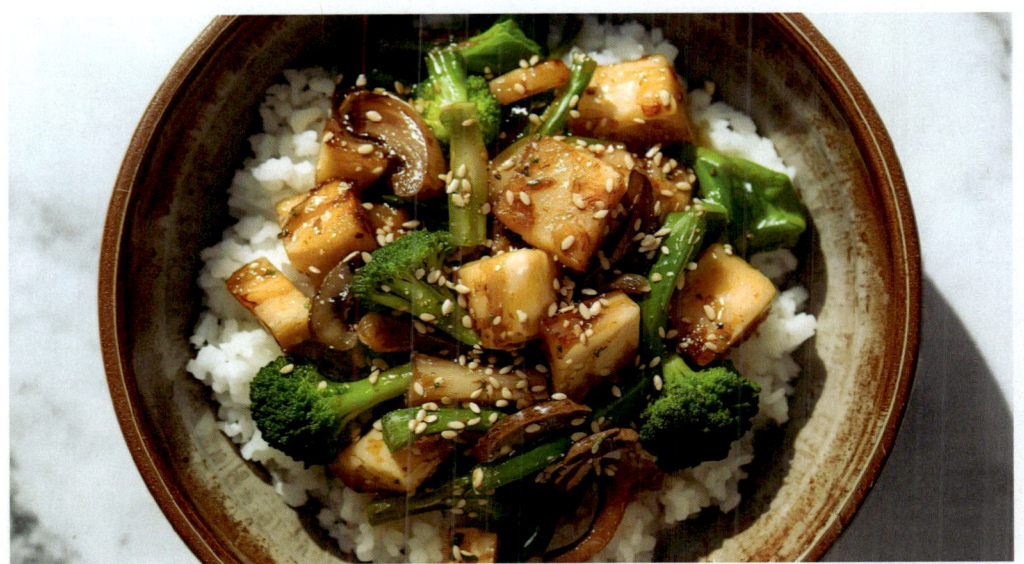

INGREDIENTS: (2 SERVINGS)

- 1 tbsp sesame oil
- 1 cup bok choy
- 1 cup broccoli
- 1 cup mushrooms
- 1 cup tofu, cubed
- 2 tbsp miso + 1 tbsp rice vinegar

INSTRUCTIONS:

- Heat oil; stir fry veggies + tofu 5 minutes.
- Add miso + vinegar; stir.
- Serve over rice.

Roasted Beet & Citrus Renewal Bowl

Mantra: "I transform through nourishment and flow."
Healing Note: Beets purify the blood and support the liver, while citrus uplifts mood and stimulates circulation.
Ancient Wisdom: Beets were used in ancient Greek and Roman cultures for vitality and detoxification — symbolizing renewal of body and spirit.

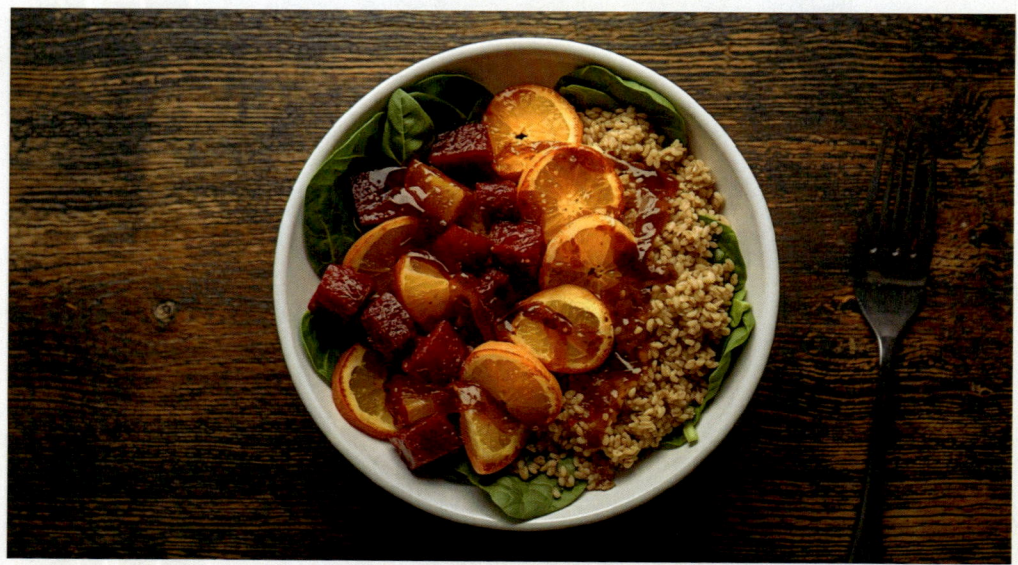

INGREDIENTS: (2 SERVINGS)

- 2 beets, roasted and cubed
- 1 orange, peeled and segmented
- 1 cup cooked farro or quinoa
- 2 cups baby spinach
- 2 tbsp olive oil
- 1 tbsp balsamic vinegar
- 1 tsp honey
- Pinch of sea salt

INSTRUCTIONS:

- Roast beets at 400°F for 35 minutes until tender; peel and cube.
- Whisk olive oil, balsamic, honey, and salt for dressing.
- Combine spinach, farro, beets, and orange segments in a bowl.
- Toss with dressing and serve warm or chilled.

Kitchari Cleansing Bowl

Mantra: "I cleanse my body and mind."
Healer's Note: Balances digestion, gently detoxifies.
Ancient Wisdom: Ayurvedic cleansing dish for thousands of years.

INGREDIENTS: (2 SERVINGS)

- 1 cup mung beans (split + soaked)
- ½ cup basmati rice
- 1 tbsp ghee or olive oil
- 1 tsp cumin seeds
- 1 tsp turmeric
- 1 tsp ginger, grated
- 6 cups water
- 2 cups spinach or kale

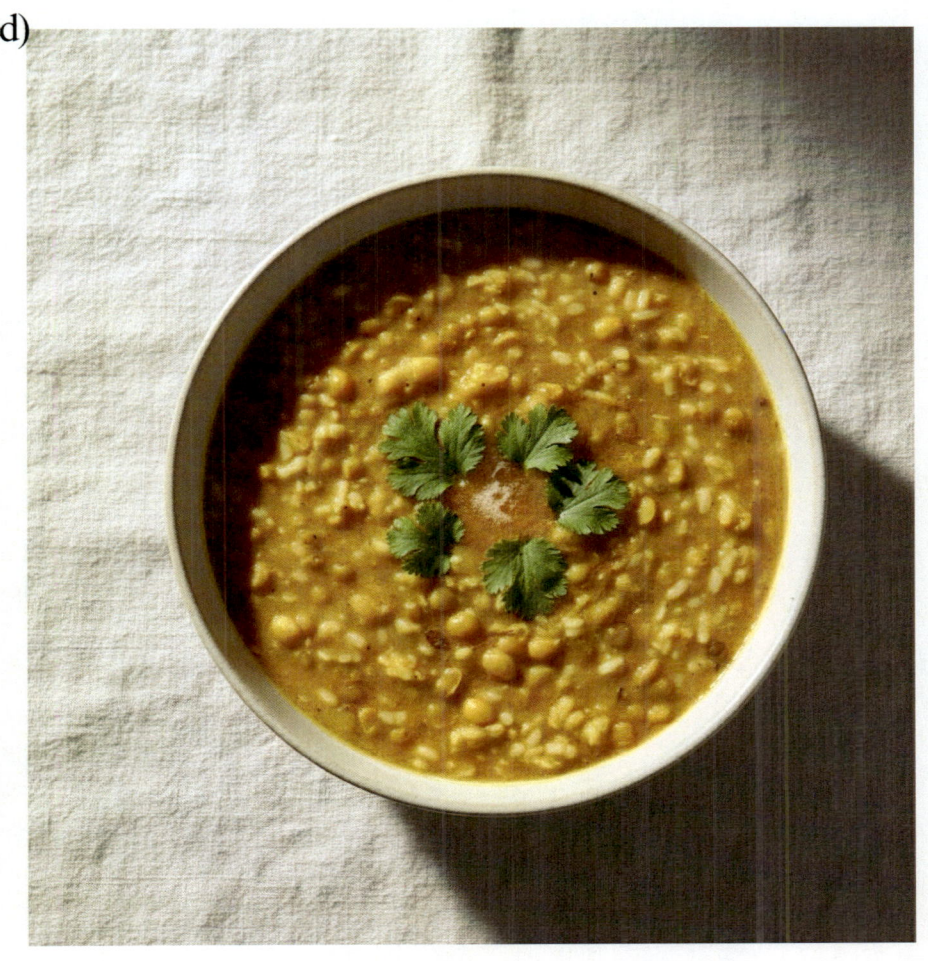

INSTRUCTIONS:

- Cook mung beans + rice with water + spices until soft. Stir in greens. Serve warm.

Chickpea Kale Salad

Mantra: "I let go of heaviness."
Healer's Note: Chickpeas fuel energy, kale cleanses the liver.
Ancient Wisdom: Greens used in spring cleanses for renewal.

INGREDIENTS: (2 SERVINGS)

- 2 cups kale, massaged with olive oil + lemon
- 1 cup chickpeas
- 1 carrot, shredded
- ½ avocado, sliced
- 2 tbsp sunflower seeds

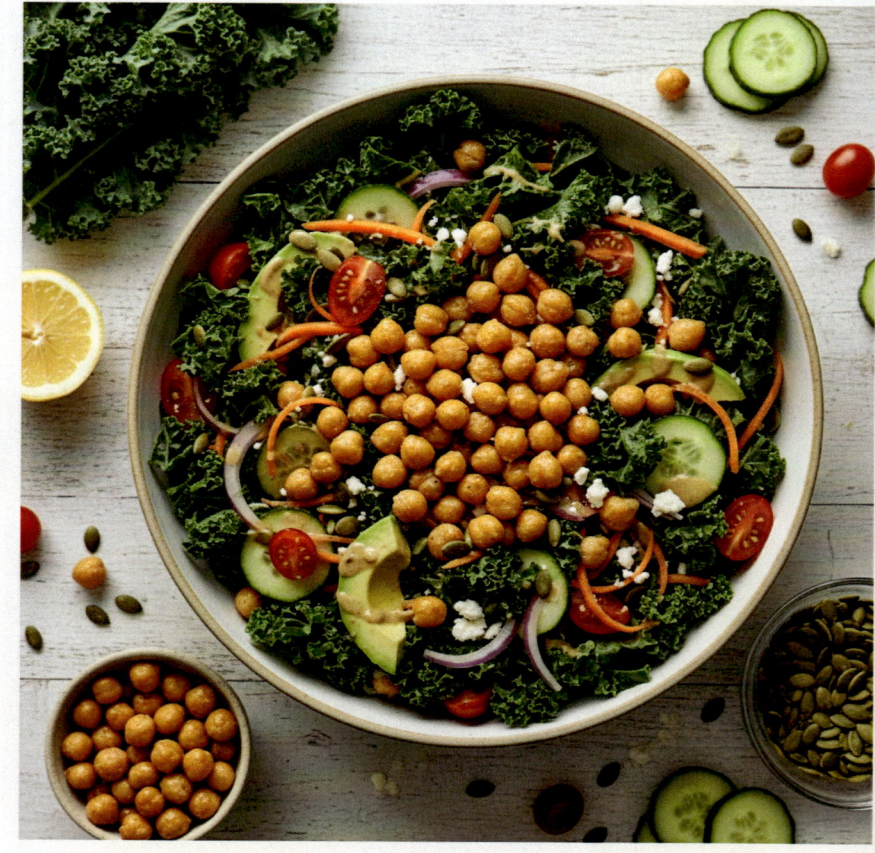

INSTRUCTIONS:

- Toss all together, season with salt + pepper.

Miso Veggie Soup

Mantra: "I embrace renewal."
Healer's Note: Miso restores gut health, mushrooms boost immunity.
Ancient Wisdom: Miso soup is a Japanese tradition for longevity.

INGREDIENTS: (4 SERVINGS)

- 4 cups water
- 3 tbsp miso paste
- 1 cup bok choy
- 1 cup mushrooms, sliced
- ½ block tofu, cubed
- 1 scallion, chopped

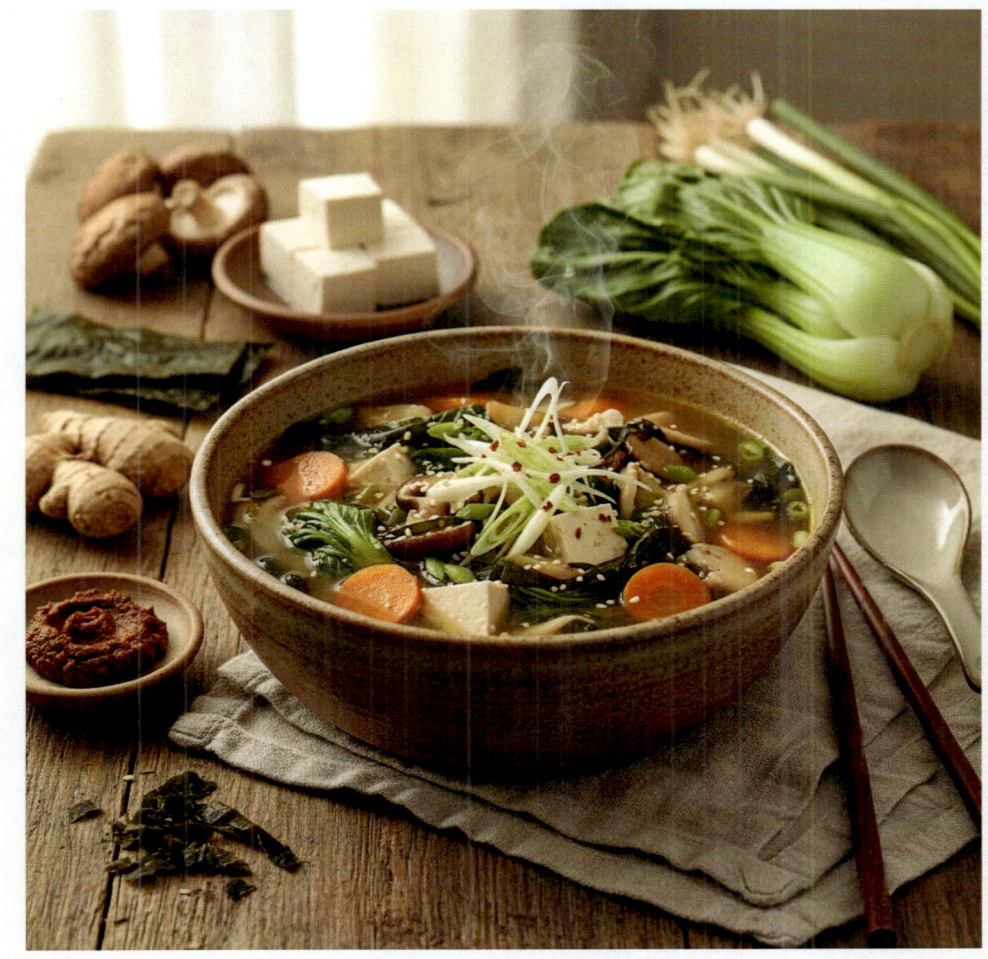

INSTRUCTIONS:

- Heat water, stir in miso. Add veggies + tofu,
  .simmer 5–10 min.

Cleansing Green Detox Salad

Mantra: "I release what weighs me down and welcome renewal."
Healing Note: Kale and parsley cleanse the liver; lemon and ginger refresh digestion.
Ancient Wisdom: Greens have symbolized renewal and spring in many cultures; parsley was sacred in Ancient Greece as a plant of cleansing and rebirth.

INGREDIENTS: (2 SERVINGS)

- 2 cups chopped kale or mixed greens
- 1 cup cucumber, diced
- 1 cup shredded carrot
- ½ cup fresh parsley or cilantro, chopped
- ½ avocado, cubed
- 2 tbsp pumpkin seeds
- Lemon-Herb Dressing
- Juice of 1 lemon
- 2 tbsp olive oil
- 1 tsp grated fresh ginger
- Pinch salt & pepper

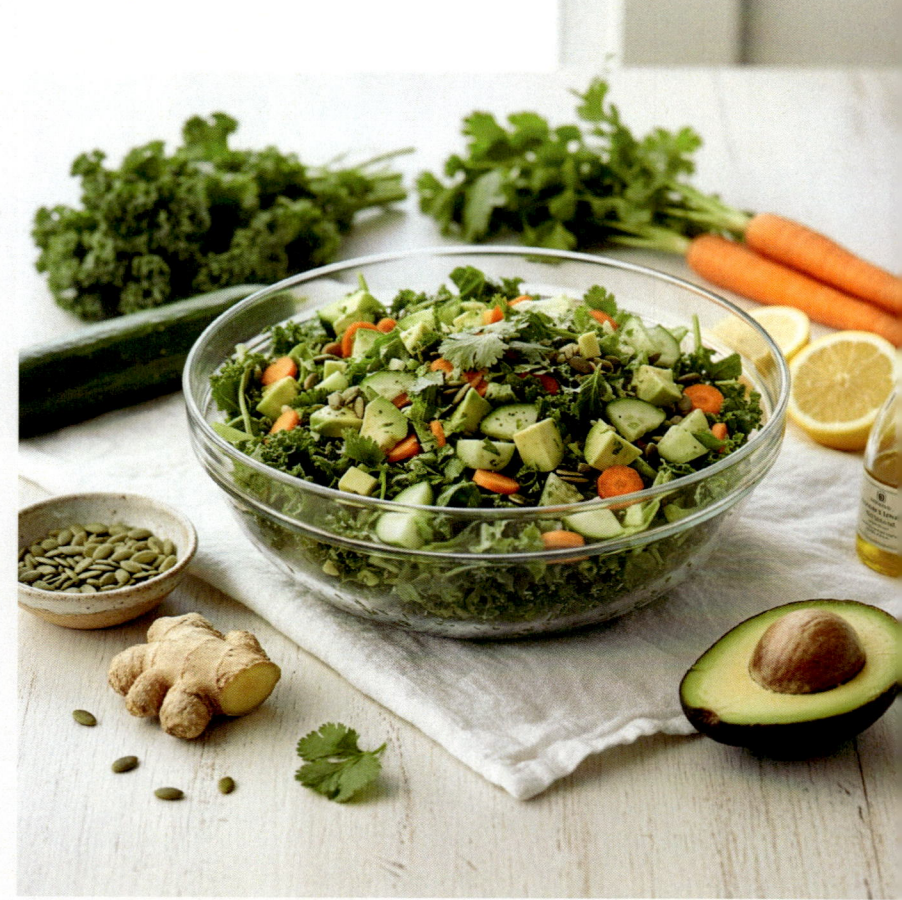

INSTRUCTIONS:

- Place kale, cucumber, carrot, parsley, and avocado in a large bowl.
- Whisk together lemon, olive oil, ginger, salt, and pepper.
- Toss salad with dressing, top with pumpkin seeds, and serve fresh.

Cleansing Cucumber & Green Apple Salad

Mantra: "I release the old and welcome renewal."
Healing Note: Cucumber cools and hydrates the body, while green apple refreshes digestion and clears stagnation. Ancient Wisdom: Apples have long symbolized new beginnings and clarity; cucumbers represented cleansing and balance in ancient Eastern medicine.

INGREDIENTS: (2 SERVINGS)

- 1 cucumber, thinly sliced
- 1 green apple, thinly sliced
- 2 cups arugula or mixed greens
- 1 tbsp olive oil
- Juice of ½ lemon
- 1 tsp honey or maple syrup
- 1 tbsp pumpkin seeds

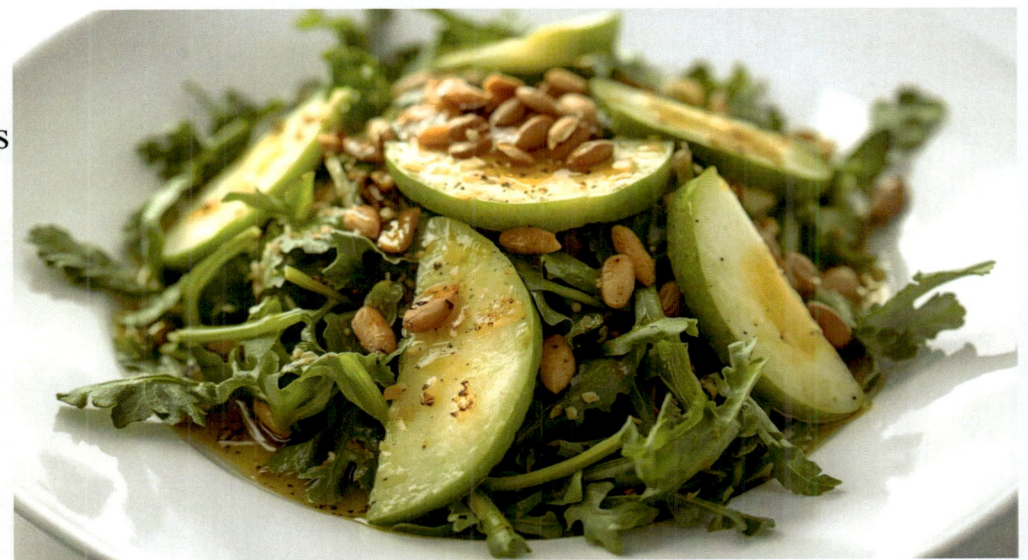

INSTRUCTIONS:

- Whisk olive oil, lemon juice, and honey into a light dressing.
- Toss cucumber, apple, and greens together.
- Sprinkle with pumpkin seeds and drizzle dressing before serving.

Zucchini Noodle Glow Bowl

Mantra: "I grow lighter, freer, and stronger each day."
Healing Note: Zucchini hydrates; miso supports gut health; edamame provides clean protein.
Ancient Wisdom: In Japan, miso soup has been eaten daily for centuries as a ritual of balance, healing, and longevity.

INGREDIENTS: (2 SERVINGS)

- 2 medium zucchini, spiralized into noodles
- 1 cup cherry tomatoes, halved
- 1 cup edamame or green peas, cooked
- 1 cup baby spinach
- 2 tbsp sesame seeds
- Light Miso-Ginger Dressing
- 2 tbsp miso paste
- 1 tbsp rice vinegar or lemon juice
- 1 tsp fresh ginger, grated
- 2 tbsp warm water (to thin)

INSTRUCTIONS:

- Spiralize zucchini into noodles. Lightly steam or serve raw for crunch.
- Arrange zucchini noodles in bowls, top with tomatoes, edamame, and spinach.
- Whisk miso, vinegar, ginger, and water until smooth.
- Drizzle dressing, sprinkle sesame seeds, and serve.

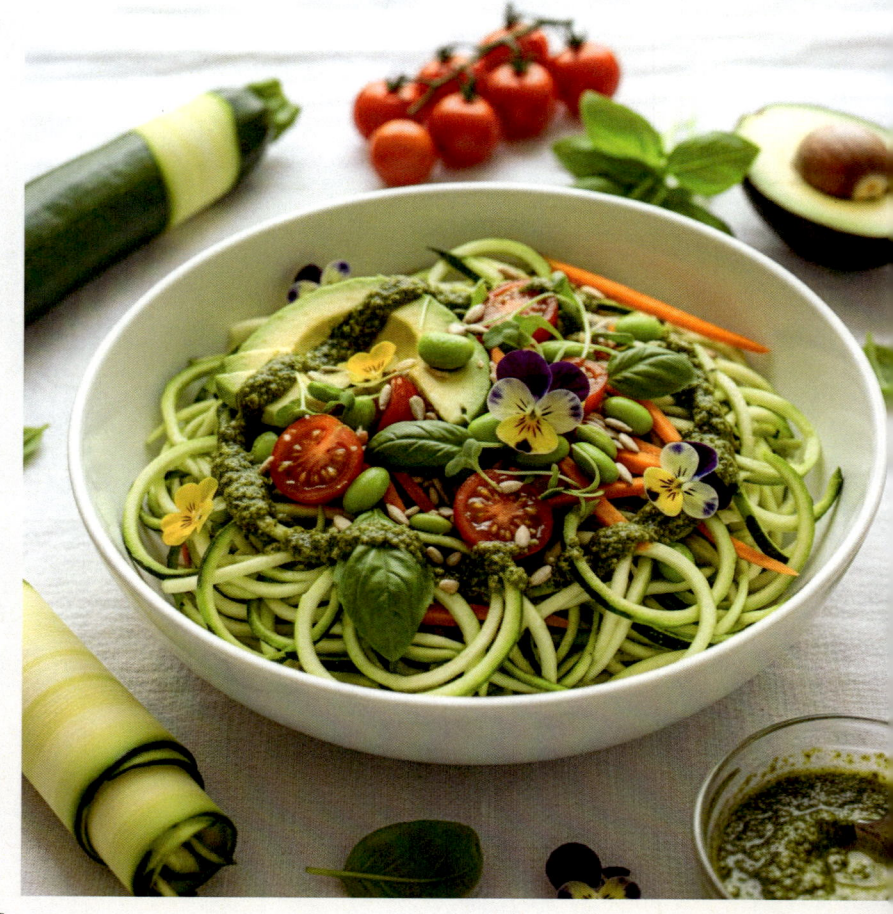

Ginger-Lemon Renewal Elixir

Mantra: "I release the old and welcome renewal."
Healing Note: Ginger stimulates circulation and digestion; lemon cleanses; mint refreshes and calms.
Ancient Wisdom: In Ayurveda and traditional healing, ginger and lemon have long been used to cleanse the body of stagnant energy, while mint symbolized breath, clarity, and renewal.

INGREDIENTS: (2 GLASSES)

- 3 cups water
- 1-inch piece fresh ginger, sliced
- Juice of 1 lemon
- 1 tsp raw honey or maple (optional)
- 4–5 fresh mint leaves

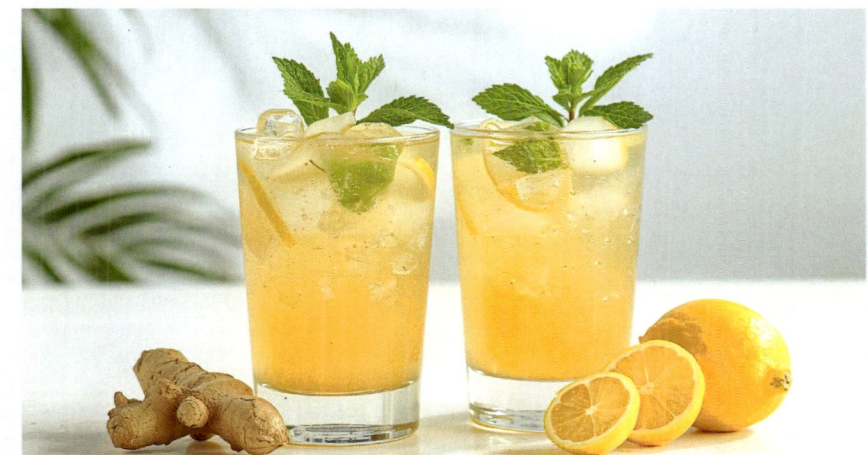

INSTRUCTIONS:

- Simmer ginger slices in water for 10 minutes.
- Strain and let cool slightly.
- Stir in lemon juice and sweetener (if using).
- Add mint leaves and let steep 2 minutes before serving.
- Enjoy warm or chilled over ice.

Green Renewal Matcha Latte

Mantra: "I rise renewed."
Healing Note: Matcha energizes; vanilla calms.
Ancient Wisdom: Tea ceremonies honored presence and renewal.

INGREDIENTS: (2 MUGS)

- 2 tsp matcha powder
- 2 cups oat milk
- 1 tsp honey
- ½ tsp vanilla

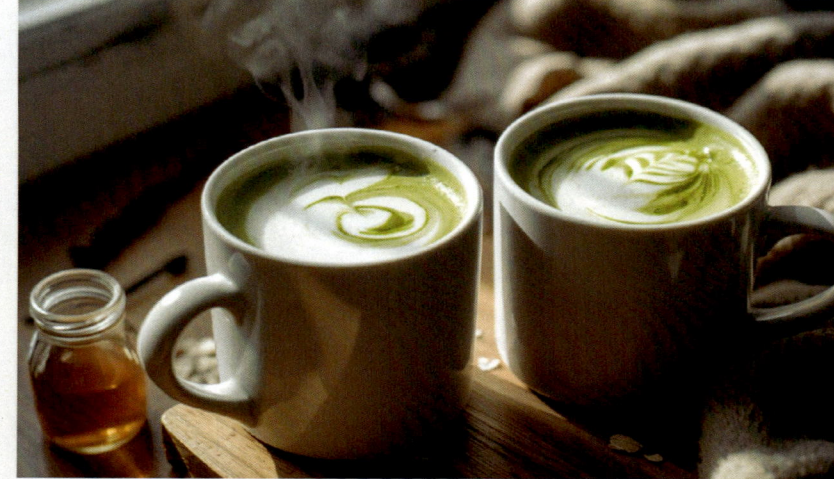

INSTRUCTIONS:

- Whisk matcha with hot water to smooth.
- Heat milk, add honey + vanilla.
- Combine and serve.

Pineapple Mint Sorbet

Mantra: "I embrace lightness and flow."
Healing Note: Pineapple cleanses; mint refreshes.
Ancient Wisdom: Mint has symbolized renewal since ancient Greece.

INGREDIENTS: (4 SERVINGS)

- 3 cups frozen pineapple
- ½ cup fresh mint leaves
- Juice of 1 lime

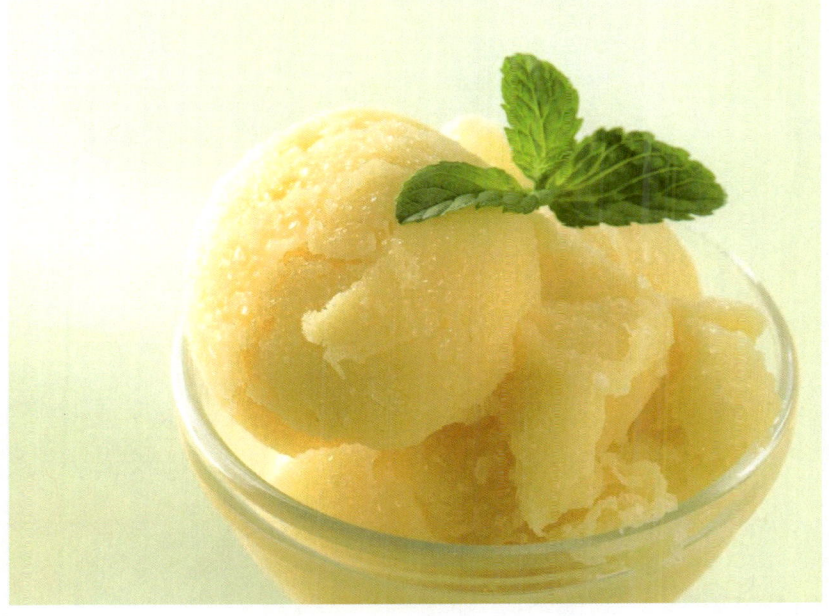

INSTRUCTIONS:

- Blend all ingredients until creamy.
- Freeze 1 hr; scoop to serve.

PILLAR 5

CONQUER
Courage, Boundaries & Strength

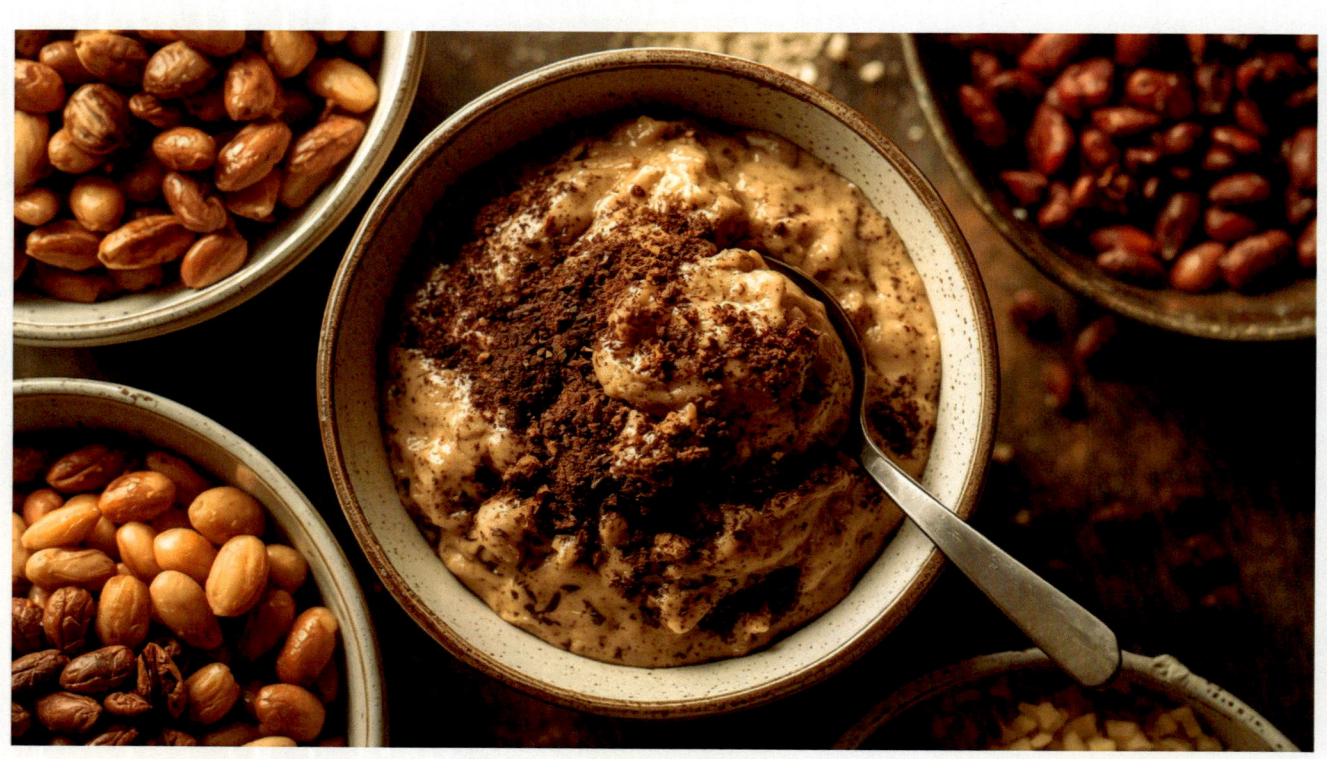

🍴 Optional Proteins & Cheeses

Conquer – Step into Power

Mantra: "I step into power with courage."
Healing Note: Strong proteins fuel resilience, stamina, and fiery confidence.
Ancient Wisdom: Warriors across cultures consumed hearty meats and bold spices before battle for strength and protection.

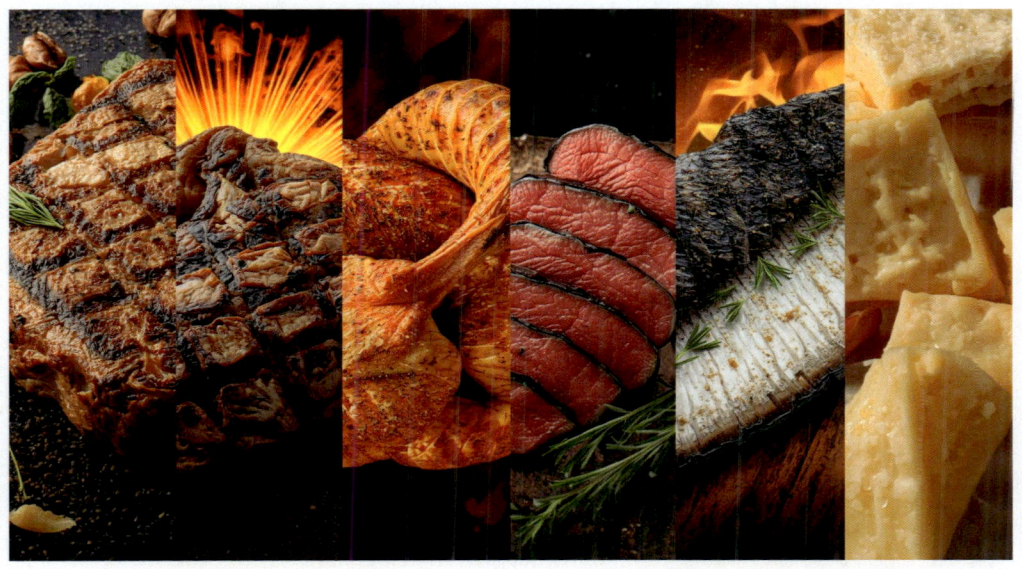

Meat (Steak): Bold, energizing, grounding.

Poultry (Spiced Chicken/Turkey): Fiery, stamina-building.

Seafood (Tuna/Swordfish): Strong flavors, commanding presence.

Cheese (Pepper Jack/Parmesan): Sharp, assertive.

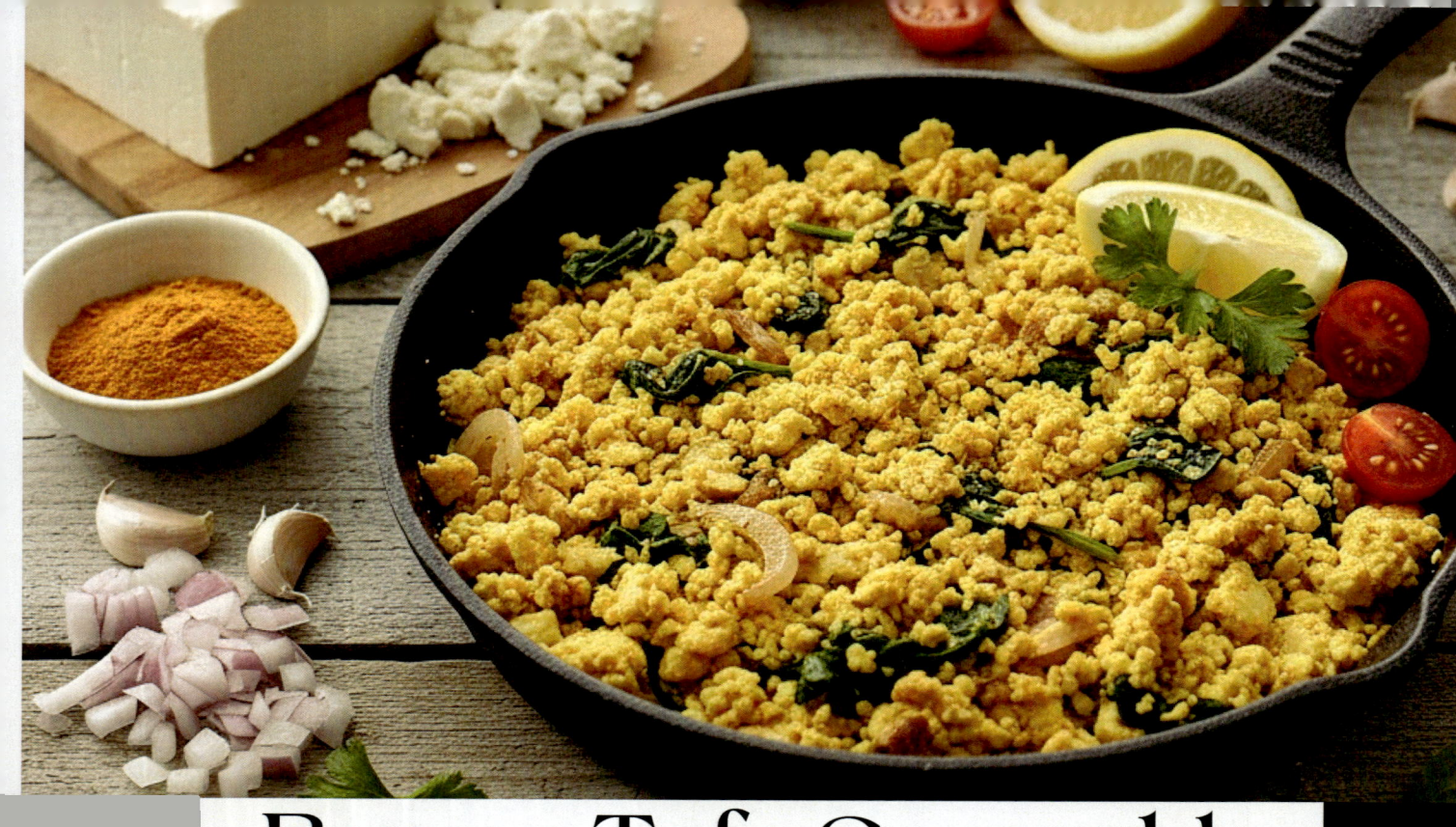

Power Tofu Scramble

Mantra: "I step into my strength."
Healing Note: Tofu fuels muscles; turmeric boosts resilience.
Ancient Wisdom: Turmeric was prized in Ayurveda for inner fire (agni) and protection.

Ingredients: (2 servings)

- 14 oz firm tofu, drained & crumbled
- 1 tbsp olive oil
- ½ onion, diced
- 1 clove garlic, minced
- 1 tsp turmeric
- 1 tbsp nutritional yeast (optional)
- 2 cups spinach
- Salt, pepper, squeeze of lemon

Instructions:

- Heat oil; sauté onion 3 minutes, add garlic 1 minute.
- Crumble in tofu, add turmeric, nutritional yeast, salt & pepper. Cook 6 minutes.
- Fold in spinach to wilt, finish with lemon.

Warrior Quinoa Power Bowl

MANTRA: "I FUEL MY BODY, I IGNITE MY STRENGTH, I STEP INTO MY POWER."

HEALING NOTE: QUINOA AND CHICKPEAS PROVIDE CLEAN PROTEIN FOR STAMINA, WHILE SWEET POTATOES AND GREENS BALANCE GROUNDING WITH ENERGY.

ANCIENT WISDOM: QUINOA WAS KNOWN AS THE "GOLD OF THE INCAS," EATEN BY WARRIORS FOR ENDURANCE. SEEDS AND GREENS WERE CARRIED AS PROTECTIVE FOODS IN TIMES OF BATTLE AND CEREMONY.

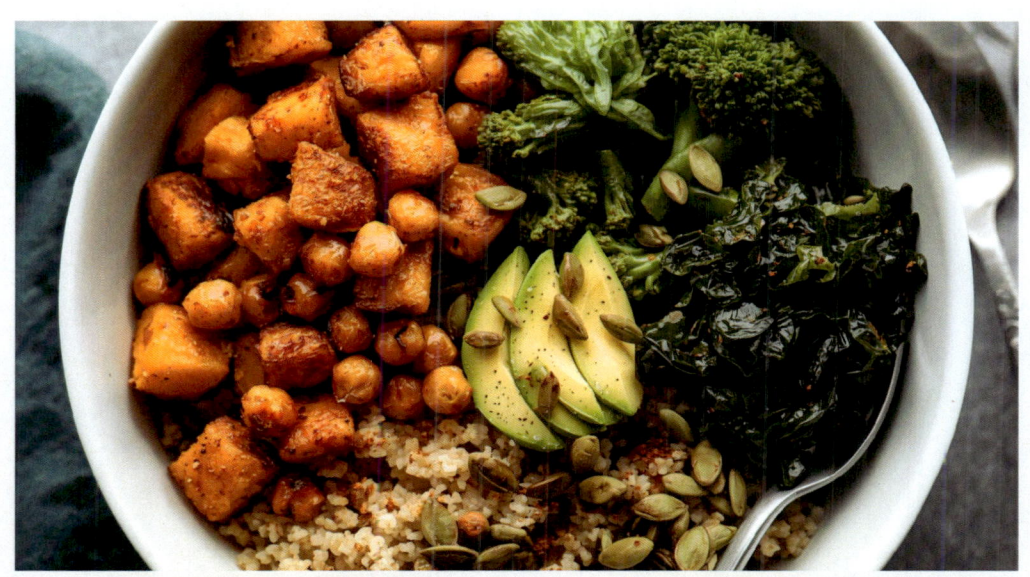

INGREDIENTS: (2 SERVINGS)

- 1 cup cooked quinoa
- 1 cup roasted sweet potato cubes
- 1 cup steamed broccoli florets
- 1 cup sautéed kale or spinach
- ½ cup roasted chickpeas (seasoned with paprika + olive oil)
- ¼ avocado, sliced
- 2 tbsp pumpkin seeds (pepitas)
- Dressing
- 2 tbsp tahini
- 1 tbsp lemon juice
- 1 tsp maple syrup
- 2–3 tbsp warm water (to thin)
- Pinch of sea salt

INSTRUCTIONS:

- Roast sweet potato cubes at 400°F for 25 minutes until golden.
- Steam broccoli until tender-crisp (about 5 minutes).
- Sauté kale/spinach in a little olive oil until just wilted.
- Roast chickpeas with paprika + olive oil at 400°F for 20 minutes until crispy.
- Assemble bowl with quinoa as base. Top with sweet potato, broccoli, greens, chickpeas, avocado slices, and pumpkin seeds.
- Whisk dressing ingredients until smooth; drizzle over bowl.

Lentil Shepherd's Pie

Mantra: "I am resilient and grounded."
Healing Note: Lentils strengthen; potatoes comfort and sustain.
Ancient Wisdom: Root vegetables have symbolized survival and stability across cultures.

INGREDIENTS: (4-5 SERVINGS)

- 2 large potatoes, boiled & mashed with olive oil + milk
- 1 tbsp olive oil
- 1 onion, diced
- 2 carrots, diced
- 1 cup lentils
- 2½ cups broth
- 1 tbsp tomato paste
- 1 tsp thyme
- 1 cup peas
- Salt & pepper

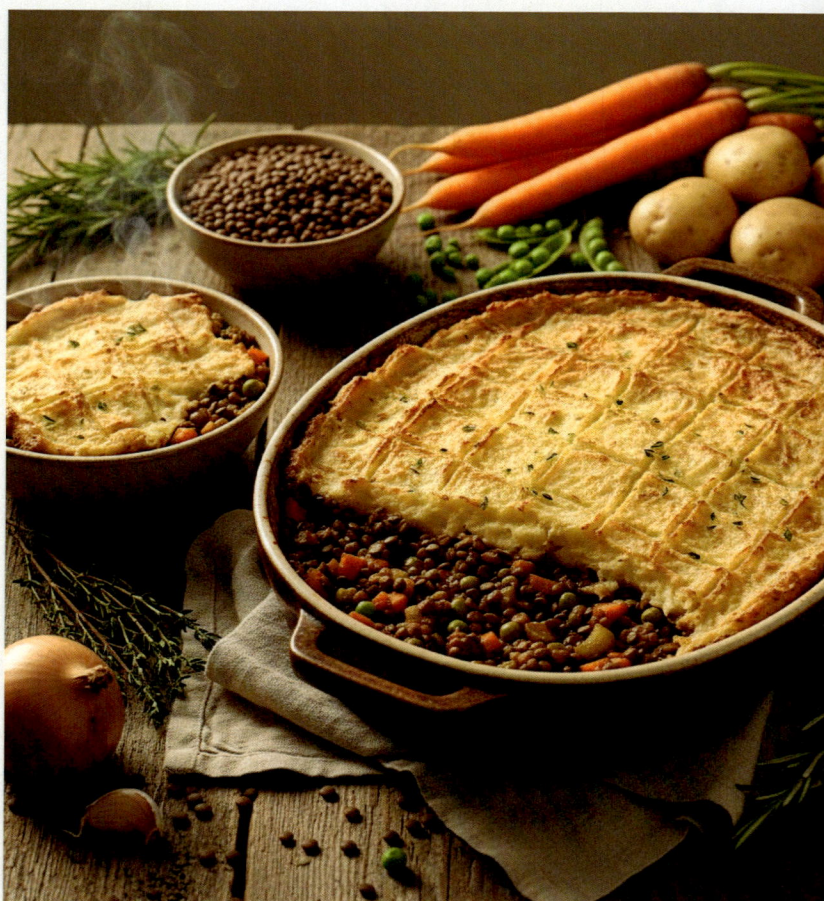

INSTRUCTIONS:

- Make mashed potatoes; set aside.
- Cook onion & carrots in oil 5 min; add lentils, broth, tomato paste, thyme. Simmer 25 min.
- Stir in peas; season.
- Spread filling in dish, top with mash. Bake at 400°F for 20 min until golden.

Spiced Red Lentil & Tomato Stew

MANTRA: "I AM STRONG, STEADY, AND UNSTOPPABLE."
HEALING NOTE: LENTILS BUILD STAMINA; TOMATOES STRENGTHEN THE HEART.
ANCIENT WISDOM: PAPRIKA AND SPICES WERE TRADED AS TREASURES, BELIEVED TO IGNITE INNER FIRE.

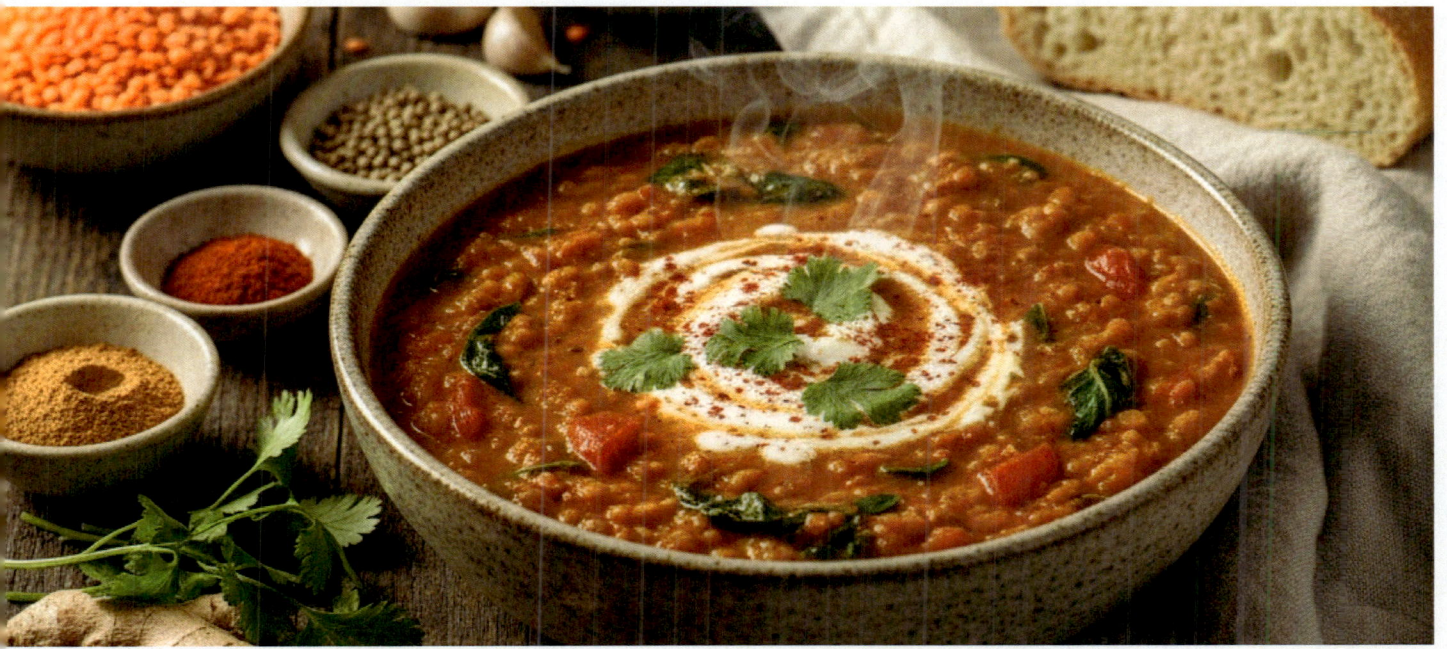

INGREDIENTS: (4 SERVINGS)

- 1 tbsp olive oil
- 1 onion, diced
- 2 cloves garlic, minced
- 1 cup red lentils, rinsed
- 1 can (14 oz) crushed tomatoes
- 4 cups vegetable broth
- 1 tsp cumin
- 1 tsp smoked paprika
- Salt & pepper
- Fresh parsley or cilantro to garnish

INSTRUCTIONS:

- Heat oil; sauté onion and garlic until fragrant.
- Add lentils, tomatoes, broth, and spices. Bring to boil, reduce heat, simmer 25 minutes.
- Adjust seasoning; garnish with fresh herbs.

Chickpea Curry

MANTRA: "I NOURISH COURAGE."
HEALER'S NOTE: CURRY SPICES BOOST METABOLISM, CHICKPEAS FUEL STRENGTH.
ANCIENT WISDOM: CURRY BLENDS HAVE BEEN USED IN AYURVEDA FOR CENTURIES FOR RESILIENCE.

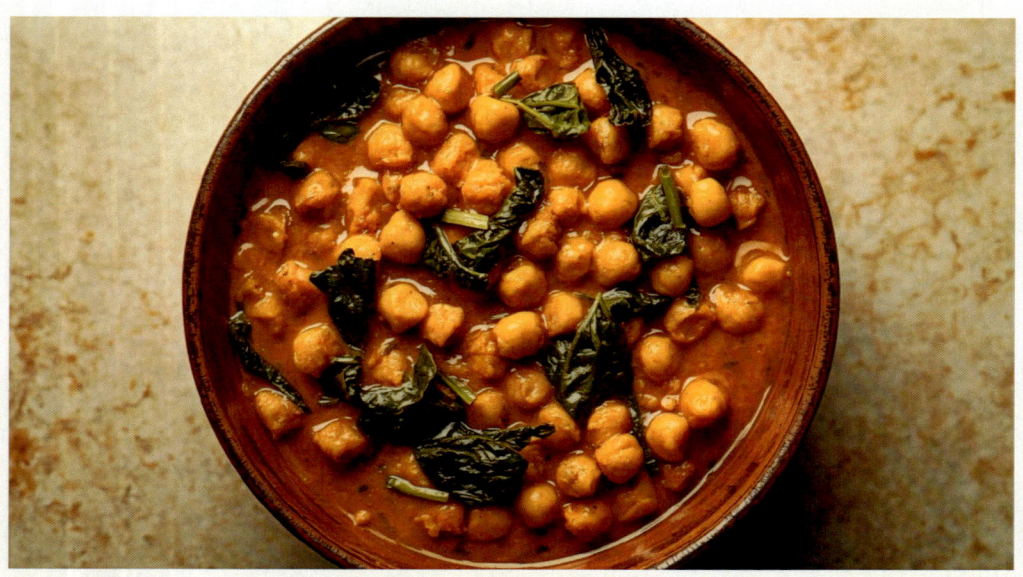

INGREDIENTS: (4 SERVINGS)

- 1 tbsp olive oil
- 1 onion, diced
- 2 cloves garlic, minced
- 1 tbsp curry powder
- 1 can coconut milk
- 1 can chickpeas, drained
- 2 cups spinach

INSTRUCTIONS:

- Heat coconut oil in a large skillet over medium heat.
- Sauté onion until translucent (about 5 minutes).
- Add garlic and ginger; cook for 1 minute until fragrant.
- Stir in curry powder; toast for 30 seconds to deepen the flavor.
- Add chickpeas, coconut milk, and tomatoes.
- Simmer gently for 15–20 minutes, stirring occasionally, until the sauce thickens.
- Stir in spinach to wilt; finish with lime juice and season to taste.
- Garnish with cilantro and serve over brown rice or quinoa.

Smoky Tempeh & Veggie Skillet

MANTRA: "I FUEL MY INNER WARRIOR."

HEALING NOTE: TEMPEH IS RICH IN PROTEIN AND PROBIOTICS; SMOKY SPICES EMPOWER CONFIDENCE.

ANCIENT WISDOM: FERMENTED FOODS LIKE TEMPEH HAVE BEEN HONORED IN ASIA FOR STRENGTH AND VITALITY.

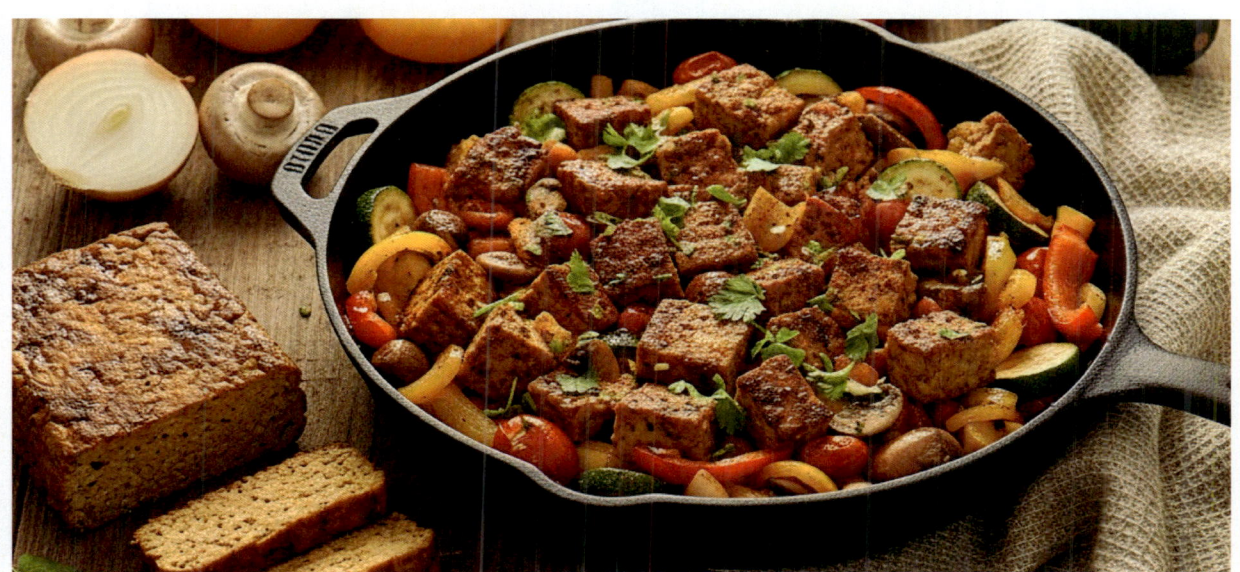

INGREDIENTS: (2 SERVINGS)

- 8 oz tempeh, cubed
- 1 tbsp olive oil
- 1 red bell pepper, sliced
- 1 zucchini, sliced
- 1 red onion, sliced
- 2 tbsp tamari or soy sauce
- 1 tsp smoked paprika
- 1 tsp garlic powder

INSTRUCTIONS:

- Heat oil in skillet; cook tempeh until golden.
- Add veggies, tamari, and spices; sauté 6–8 minutes until tender.
- Serve hot with quinoa or rice.

Spicy Black Bean Tacos

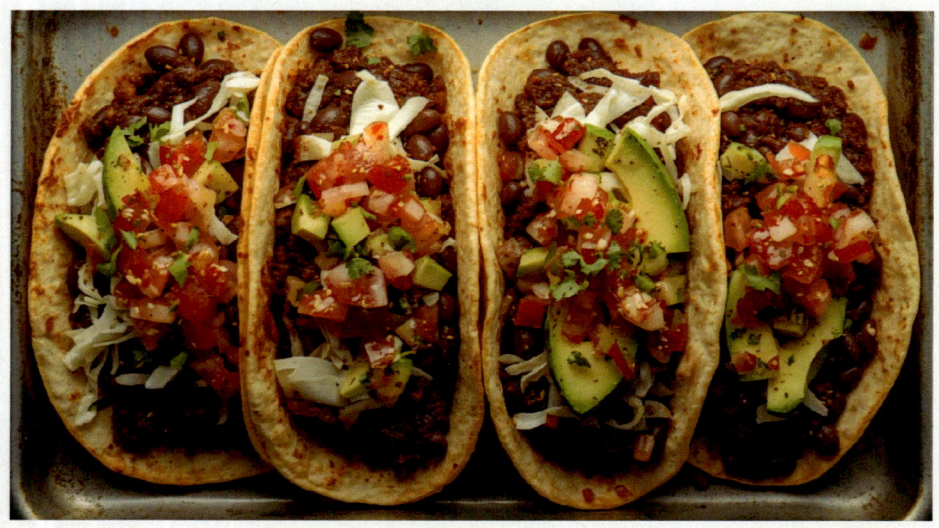

INGREDIENTS: (2 SERVINGS)

- 4 corn tortillas (or whole-grain if preferred)
- 1 can (15 oz) black beans, drained and rinsed
- 1 tsp olive oil
- ½ tsp cumin
- ½ tsp smoked paprika
- ¼ tsp chili powder (or to taste)
- 1 garlic clove, minced
- Salt & pepper to taste
- 1 cup shredded purple cabbage
- ½ avocado, sliced
- ¼ cup fresh cilantro
- Juice of ½ lime
- Optional toppings:
- Salsa or pico de gallo
- Vegan sour cream or Greek yogurt
- Jalapeño slices for extra heat

INSTRUCTIONS:

- Warm olive oil in a skillet over medium heat.
- Add garlic, cumin, paprika, and chili powder; stir 30 seconds until fragrant.
- Add black beans, mashing lightly with a fork; cook 3–5 minutes until thick and warmed through.
- Season with salt, pepper, and lime juice.
- Warm tortillas, then fill with spiced beans, cabbage, avocado, and cilantro.
- Add desired toppings and serve immediately.

Bold Spiced Chickpea & Spinach Curry

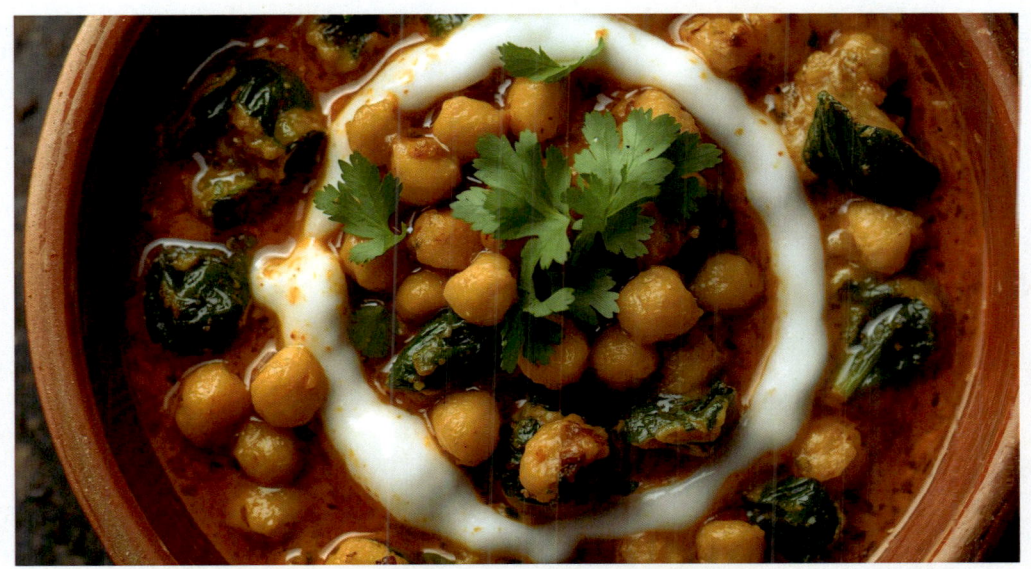

INGREDIENTS: (2 SERVINGS)

- 1 tbsp coconut oil
- 1 onion, diced
- 2 garlic cloves
- 1 tbsp curry powder
- 1 can chickpeas
- 1 cup diced tomatoes
- 2 cups spinach

INSTRUCTIONS:

- Cook onion + garlic.
- Add curry powder, tomatoes, chickpeas. Simmer 10 min.
- Stir in spinach.

Black Bean Quinoa Bowl

MANTRA: "I FUEL MY STRENGTH."
HEALER'S NOTE: QUINOA + BEANS PROVIDE COMPLETE PROTEIN.
ANCIENT WISDOM: BEANS + CORN WERE STAPLES OF SURVIVAL IN INDIGENOUS TRADITIONS.

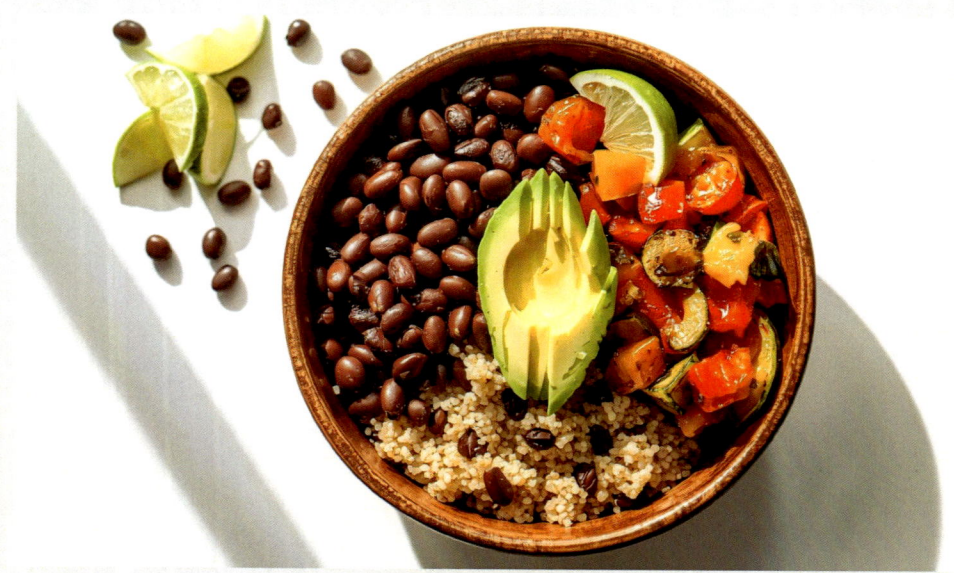

INGREDIENTS: (2 SERVINGS)

- 1 cup cooked quinoa
- 1 cup cooked black beans (or canned, rinsed and drained)
- ½ avocado, sliced
- 1 cup roasted corn (fresh or frozen)
- 1 cup cherry tomatoes, halved
- 1 tbsp olive oil
- Juice of 1 lime
- 2 tbsp chopped cilantro
- Pinch of sea salt and pepper
- Optional: sliced jalapeño or chili flakes for heat

INSTRUCTIONS:

- In a large bowl, layer quinoa, black beans, corn, and tomatoes.
- Add sliced avocado and cilantro on top.
- Drizzle with olive oil and lime juice.
- Season with salt, pepper, and chili flakes if desired.
- Toss gently and serve warm or chilled.

Power Greens & Bean Salad

INGREDIENTS: (2 SERVINGS)

- 2 cups kale, massaged with olive oil & lemon
- 1 cup black beans
- 1 cup roasted sweet potato cubes
- ½ avocado, sliced
- 2 tbsp pumpkin seeds
- Dressing: 2 tbsp tahini, juice of ½ lemon, 1–2 tbsp water, salt, pepper

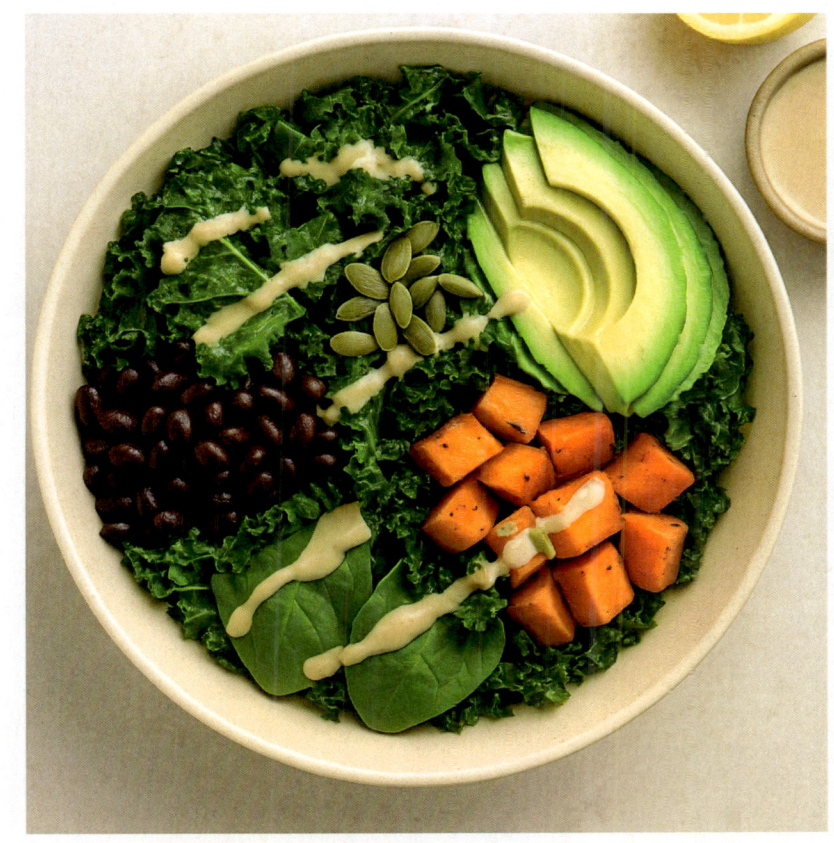

INSTRUCTIONS:

- Heat oil in skillet; cook tempeh until golden.
- Add veggies, tamari, and spices; sauté 6–8 minutes until tender.
- Serve hot with quinoa or rice.

Fiery Golden Turmeric Tonic

Mantra: "I ignite my inner fire."
Healing Note: Turmeric heals; cayenne awakens courage.
Ancient Wisdom: Fire-tonics were used as protective potions.

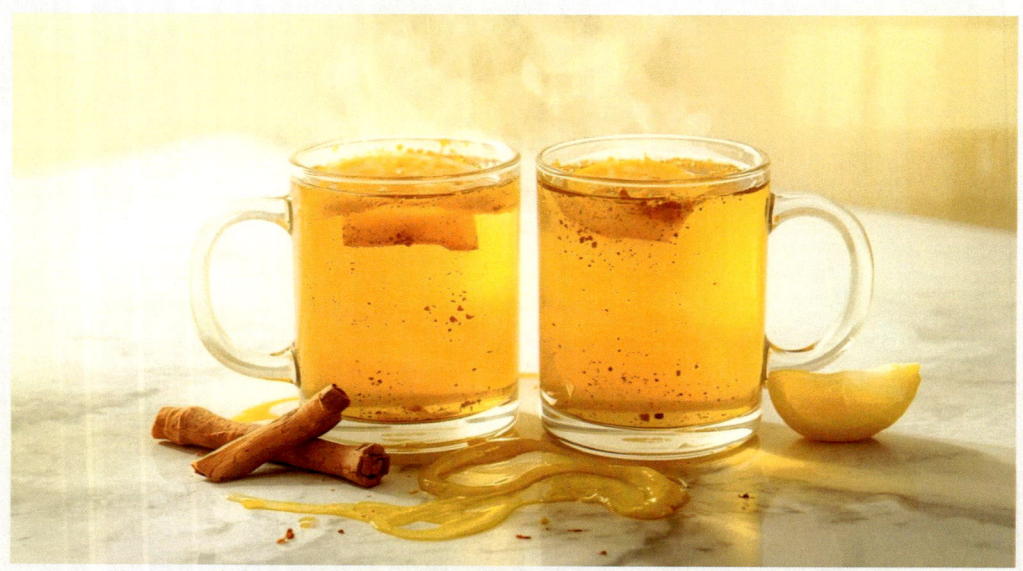

INGREDIENTS: (2 MUGS)

- 2 cups warm water
- ½ tsp turmeric
- 1 pinch cayenne
- 1 tsp lemon juice
- 1 tsp honey

INSTRUCTIONS:

- Stir all ingredients in warm water.
- Sip slowly.

Power Green Smoothie

Mantra: "I awaken my energy and move through the day with clarity and light."
Healing Note: This smoothie is a powerhouse for cleansing and renewal. Spinach oxygenates the blood, ginger boosts metabolism, and apple and lemon flush the liver. Together, they energize the body, refresh the mind, and awaken intuitive awareness.
Ancient Wisdom: Greens have long symbolized renewal and life force. In many ancient cultures, early spring greens were among the first foods harvested — representing rebirth, balance, and connection to the Earth's awakening energy.

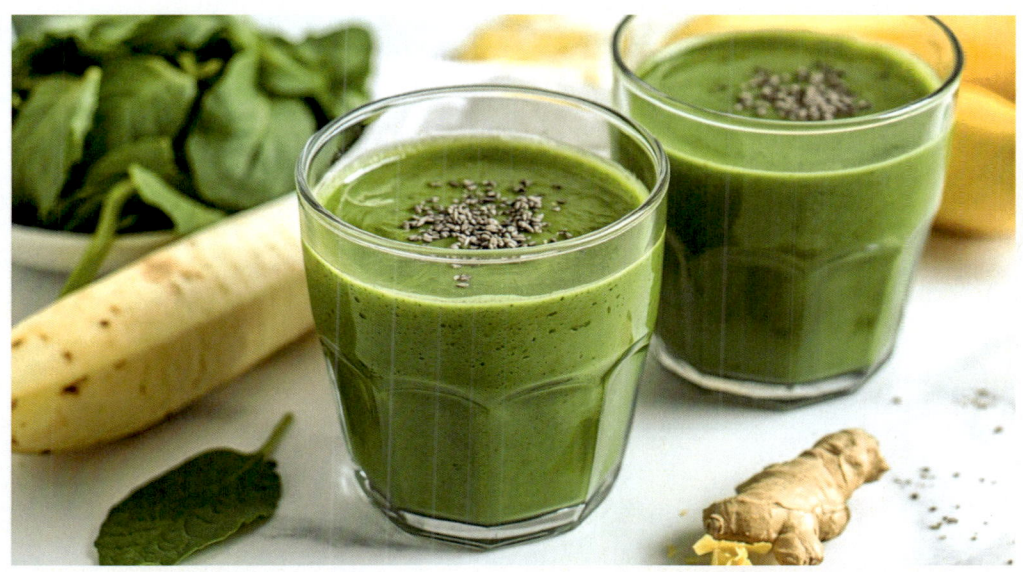

INGREDIENTS: (2 GLASSES)

- 2 cups fresh spinach (or kale for a deeper flavor)
- 1 green apple, cored and sliced
- ½ banana (for creaminess)
- 1 small cucumber, peeled and chopped
- 1 tbsp fresh lemon juice
- 1-inch piece fresh ginger (or ½ tsp grated)
- 1 cup coconut water (or filtered water for lighter taste)
- 1 tbsp chia seeds (optional for extra energy)
- 3–4 ice cubes (optional for a chilled, refreshing version)

INSTRUCTIONS:

- Add all ingredients to a blender, starting with the liquid base.
- Blend on high until smooth and vibrant green.
- Taste and adjust — add a splash more lemon for brightness or a bit of banana for sweetness.
- Pour into glasses and enjoy immediately to capture the fresh enzymes and nutrients.

Warrior's Cacao Ritual Drink

MANTRA: "I DRINK IN COURAGE AND STRENGTH."
HEALING NOTE: CACAO OPENS THE HEART; CAYENNE STIRS VITALITY.
ANCIENT WISDOM: AZTEC WARRIORS DRANK CACAO MIXED WITH SPICE BEFORE BATTLE.

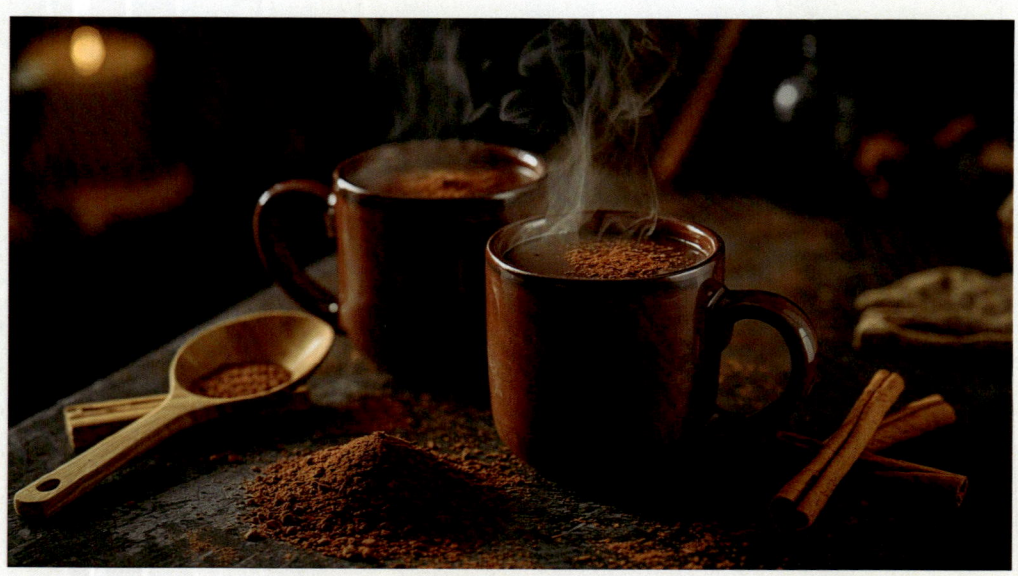

INGREDIENTS: (2 MUGS)

- 2 cups oat milk
- 2 tbsp raw cacao powder
- ½ tsp cinnamon
- Pinch of cayenne
- 1 tsp honey or maple syrup

INSTRUCTIONS:

- Heat oat milk.
- Whisk in cacao, cinnamon, and cayenne.
- Sweeten to taste.

Dark Cacao Chili Truffles

Mantra: "I taste the strength of courage."
Healing Note: Cacao + chili fuel bravery.
Ancient Wisdom: The Aztecs paired cacao + chili in warrior rituals.

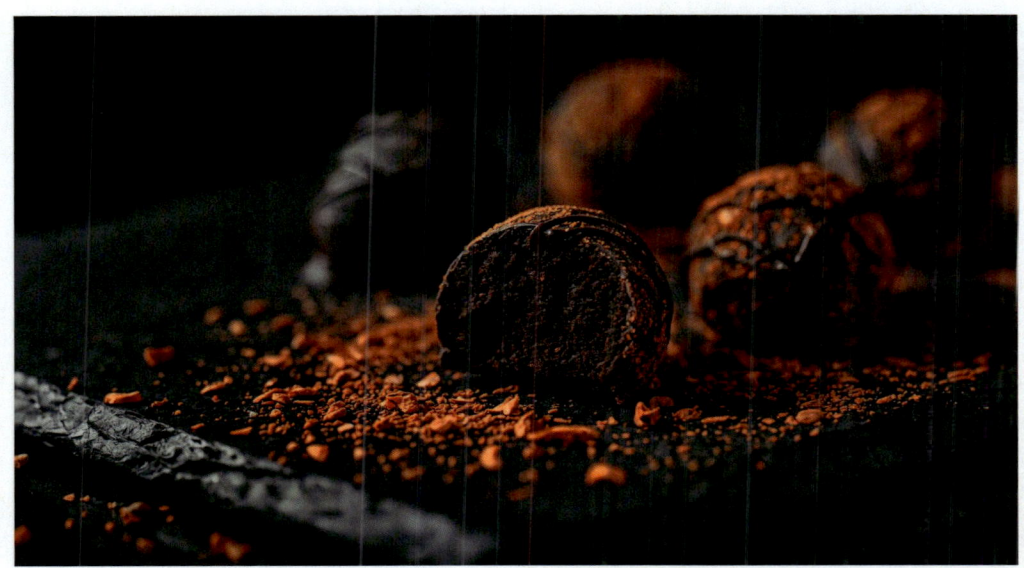

Ingredients: (12 truffles)

- 1 cup dates
- ½ cup almonds
- 3 tbsp cacao
- 1 tsp cayenne
- 2 tbsp almond butter

Instructions:

- Blend ingredients until sticky.
- Roll into balls; dust with cacao.
- Chill before serving.

Cacao Energy Bliss Balls

Mantra: "I energize my body with joy."
Healing Note: Dates give quick natural energy; cacao elevates mood and focus.
Ancient Wisdom: Nuts and seeds have been carried for centuries as symbols of strength and vitality.

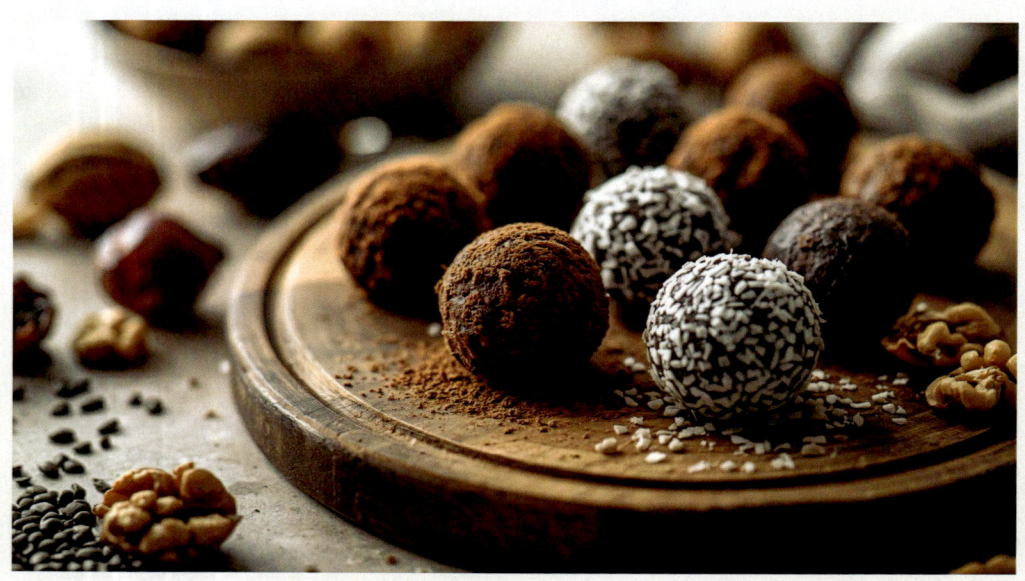

Ingredients: (12 balls)

- 1 cup pitted dates
- ½ cup walnuts or almonds
- ¼ cup raw cacao powder
- 2 tbsp chia or flax seeds
- 1 tsp vanilla extract
- Pinch sea salt
- (Optional) shredded coconut or extra cacao for rolling

Instructions:

- In a food processor, pulse the nuts until finely ground.
- Add dates, cacao, chia/flax, vanilla, and salt. Blend until mixture becomes sticky.
- Scoop about 1 tbsp at a time and roll between your palms to form balls.
- (Optional) Roll balls in shredded coconut or dust with cacao.
- Place on a tray and refrigerate for at least 1 hour before serving.

PILLAR 6

EMBODY
Integration &
Abundance

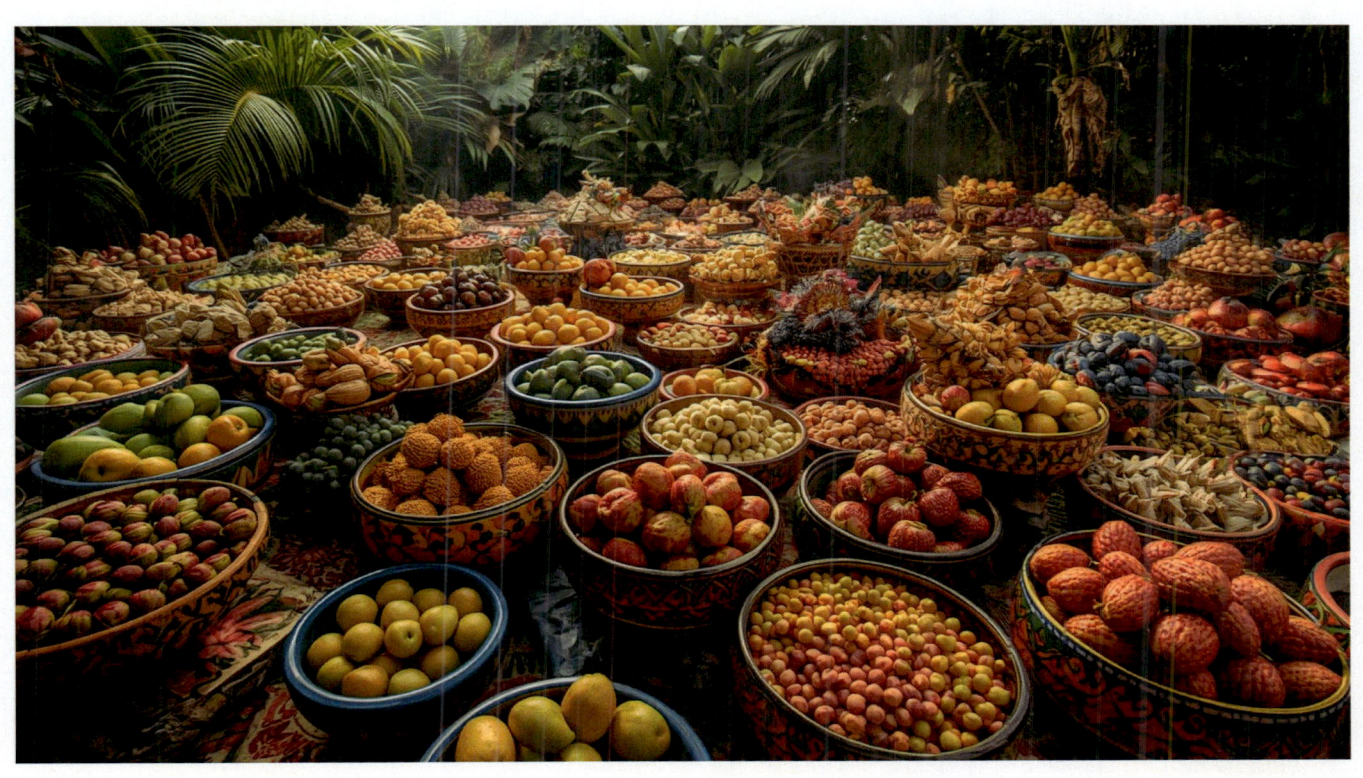

¶❙ Optional Proteins & Cheeses

Embody – Live Abundance

Mantra: "I embody joy and abundance."
Healing Note: Rich proteins paired with shared meals foster connection and celebration.
Ancient Wisdom: Feasts with luxurious foods symbolized prosperity, fertility, and communal joy in many traditions.

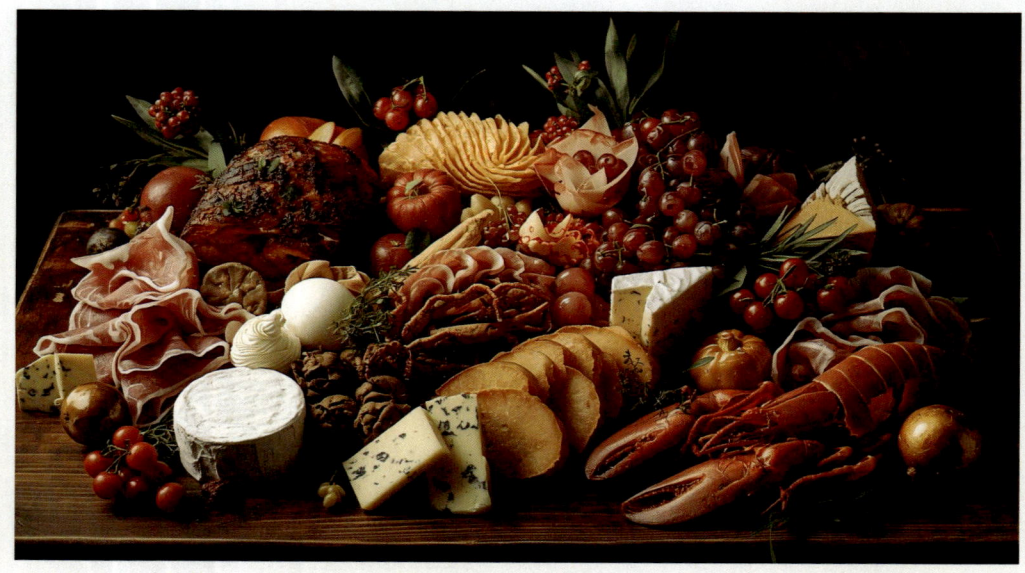

Meat (Prosciutto): Adds richness and celebratory flair.

Poultry (Roast Duck): Traditional abundance food.

Seafood (Scallops/Lobster): Luxurious, celebratory.

Cheese (Brie/Burrata/Blue): Creamy indulgence, communal sharing.

Rainbow Veggie Flatbread

MANTRA: "I EMBODY COLORFUL ABUNDANCE."
HEALING NOTE: ROASTED VEGGIES ENERGIZE; HUMMUS GROUNDS.
ANCIENT WISDOM: FLATBREADS WERE STAPLE CELEBRATORY FOODS ACROSS MIDDLE
EASTERN CULTURES.

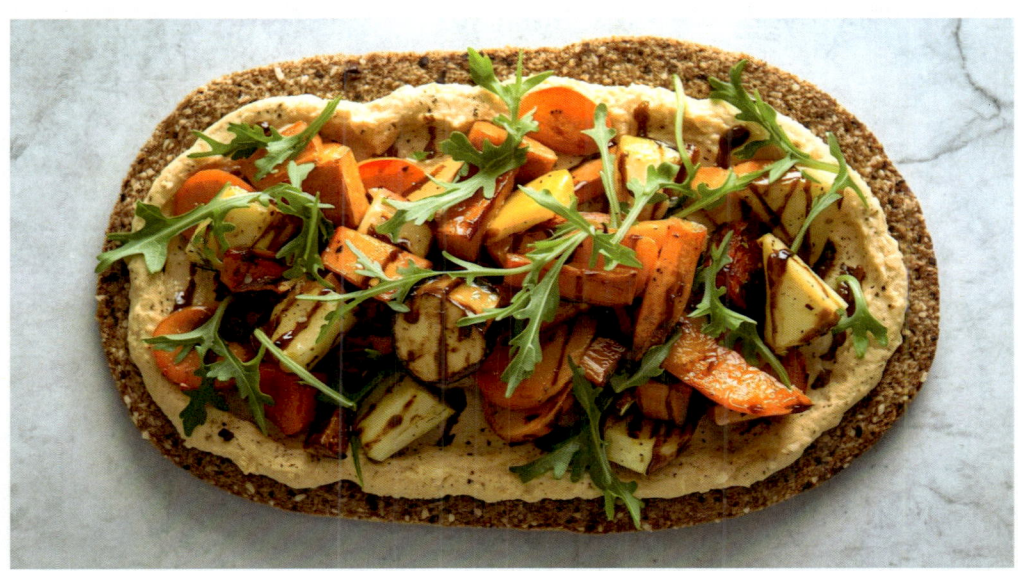

INGREDIENTS: (2 SERVINGS)

- 2 whole grain flatbreads
- 2 tbsp hummus or cashew spread
- 1 cup roasted mixed veggies
  (carrots, zucchini, peppers)
- ½ cup arugula
- Balsamic drizzle

INSTRUCTIONS:

- Spread hummus on flatbreads.
- Top with roasted veggies and arugula.
- Drizzle with balsamic, slice, and serve.

Cucumber Avocado Summer Rolls

Mantra: "I embody freshness and flow."
Healing Note: Fresh vegetables hydrate and refresh the body.
Ancient Wisdom: Rolls and wraps have symbolized abundance and prosperity in Asian feasting traditions.

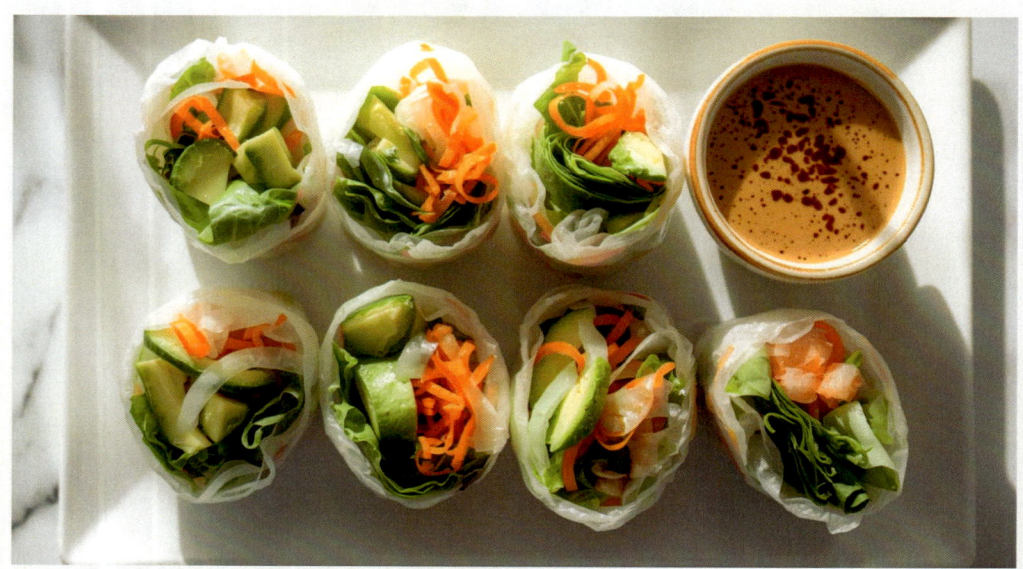

INGREDIENTS: (2 SERVINGS)

- 8 rice paper wrappers
- 1 cucumber, julienned
- 1 carrot, julienned
- ½ avocado, sliced
- 1 cup mixed greens
- Dipping sauce: 2 tbsp peanut butter + 1 tbsp tamari + warm water

INSTRUCTIONS:

- Dip rice paper in warm water to soften.
- Fill with cucumber, carrot, avocado, and greens.
- Roll tightly; serve with dipping sauce.

Tropical Pineapple Rice

Mantra: "I embody joy in every moment."
Healing Note: Pineapple uplifts mood; rice provides grounding comfort.
Ancient Wisdom: Pineapple was seen as a symbol of welcome and hospitality in many cultures.

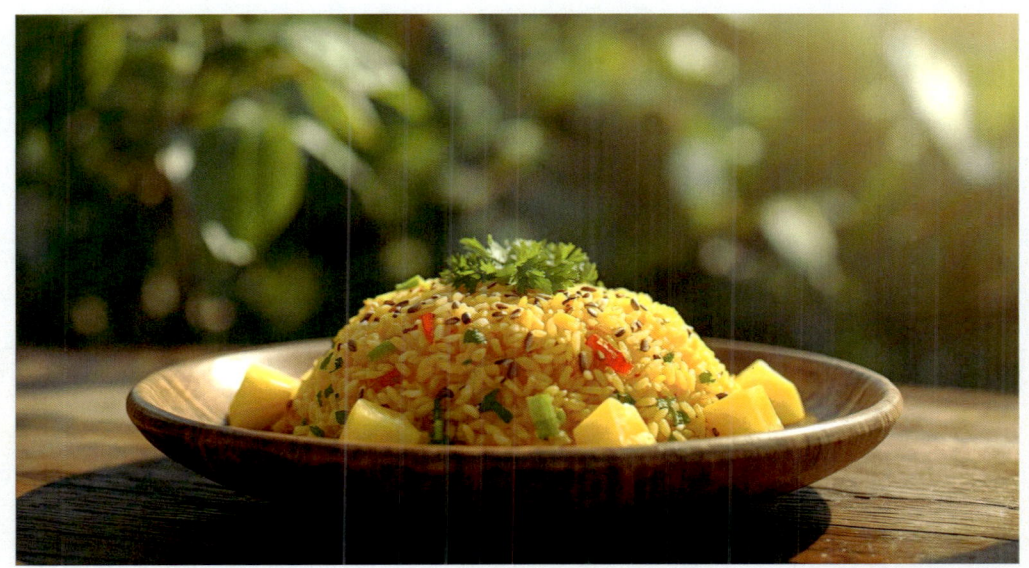

INGREDIENTS: (4 SERVINGS)

- 2 cups cooked jasmine rice
- 1 cup pineapple chunks
- 1 cup bell peppers, diced
- ½ cup peas
- 2 tbsp soy sauce or tamari
- 1 tbsp sesame oil

INSTRUCTIONS:

- Heat sesame oil; sauté peppers and peas.
- Add rice, pineapple, soy sauce; stir fry 5 minutes.
- Serve warm, garnish with scallions.

Mediterranean Stuffed Peppers

MANTRA: "I AM FILLED WITH ABUNDANCE AND JOY."
HEALING NOTE: PEPPERS ENERGIZE; QUINOA AND CHICKPEAS PROVIDE STRENGTH.
ANCIENT WISDOM: MEDITERRANEAN DIETS CENTERED ON VEGETABLES AND GRAINS AS SYMBOLS OF VITALITY.

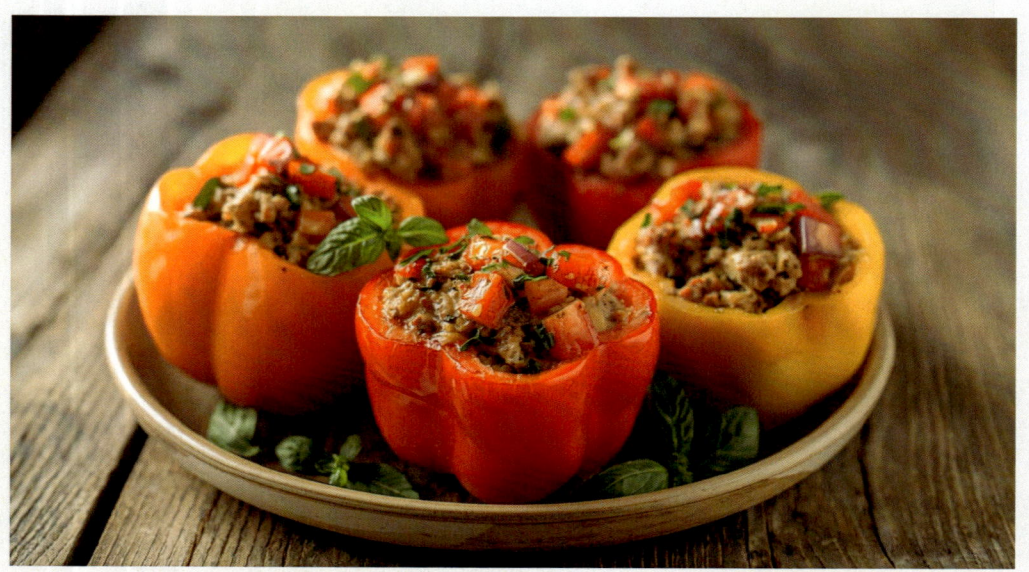

INGREDIENTS: (4 SERVINGS)

- 4 bell peppers, halved and seeded
- 1 cup cooked quinoa
- 1 cup chickpeas
- ½ cup diced tomatoes
- ¼ cup olives, chopped
- 2 tbsp olive oil, oregano, salt, pepper

INSTRUCTIONS:

- Mix quinoa, chickpeas, tomatoes, olives, oil, oregano, salt, pepper.
- Stuff mixture into peppers.
- Bake at 375°F for 25 minutes.

Lemon Basil Pasta

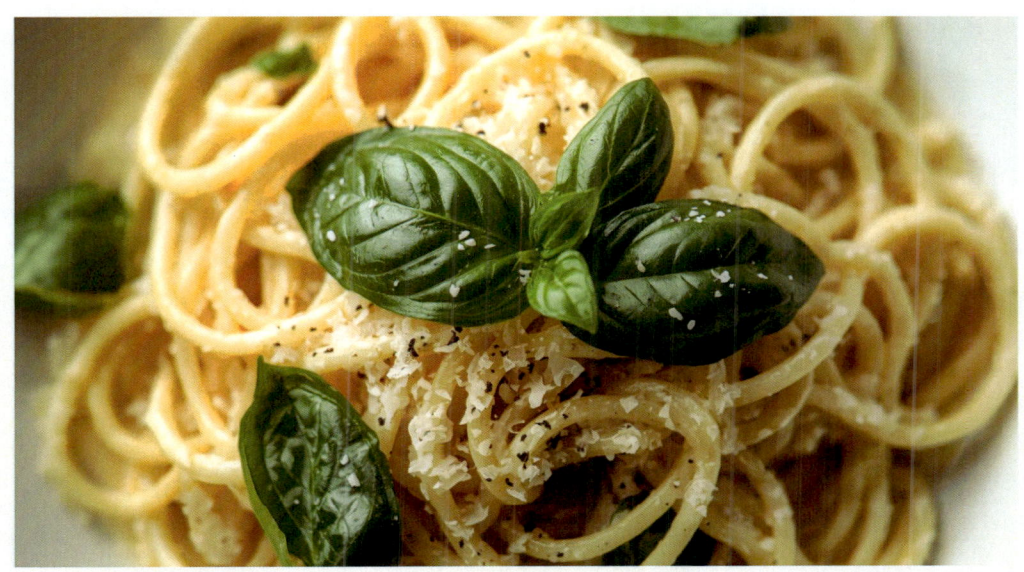

INGREDIENTS: (2 SERVINGS)

- 6 oz whole grain or gluten-free pasta
- 2 tbsp olive oil
- Zest + juice of 1 lemon
- 1 cup cherry tomatoes, halved
- 2 cups fresh basil leaves
- Salt & pepper

INSTRUCTIONS:

- Cook pasta, reserve ½ cup pasta water.
- Heat olive oil; add lemon juice, zest, tomatoes.
- Toss pasta with sauce, basil, and reserved water if needed.
- Season and serve.

Carrot & Chickpea Nourish Bowl

RITUAL: PAUSE BEFORE EATING, WHISPER: "I HONOR THE EARTH THAT NOURISHES ME."
ANCIENT WISDOM: SESAME SEEDS WERE SYMBOLS OF LONGEVITY IN ANCIENT MESOPOTAMIA.
HEALING NOTE:A DEEPLY BALANCING MEAL FOR GROUNDING AND DIGESTION. CHICKPEAS OFFER
STEADY, SUSTAINING ENERGY, WHILE CARROTS NURTURE THE SOLAR PLEXUS — THE CENTER OF
CONFIDENCE AND VITALITY. THE TAHINI DRESSING PROVIDES HEALTHY FATS TO KEEP YOU SATISFIED
AND CENTERED, TURNING A SIMPLE MEAL INTO A RITUAL OF NOURISHMENT AND INNER STEADINESS.

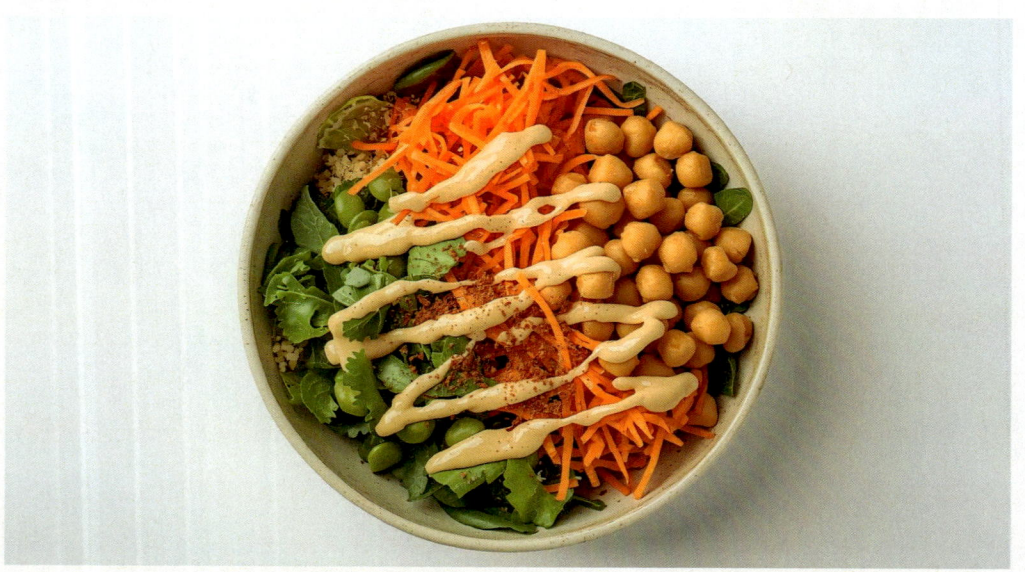

INGREDIENTS: (2 SERVINGS)

- 1 cup cooked chickpeas
- 2 carrots, shredded
- 2 cups mixed greens
- 2 tbsp tahini
- Juice of 1 lemon
- 1 tsp garlic powder
- Water to thin

INSTRUCTIONS:

- Arrange greens, carrots, and chickpeas in bowl.
- Whisk tahini, lemon juice, garlic powder, water until creamy.
- Drizzle dressing over bowl.

Rainbow Nourish Bowl

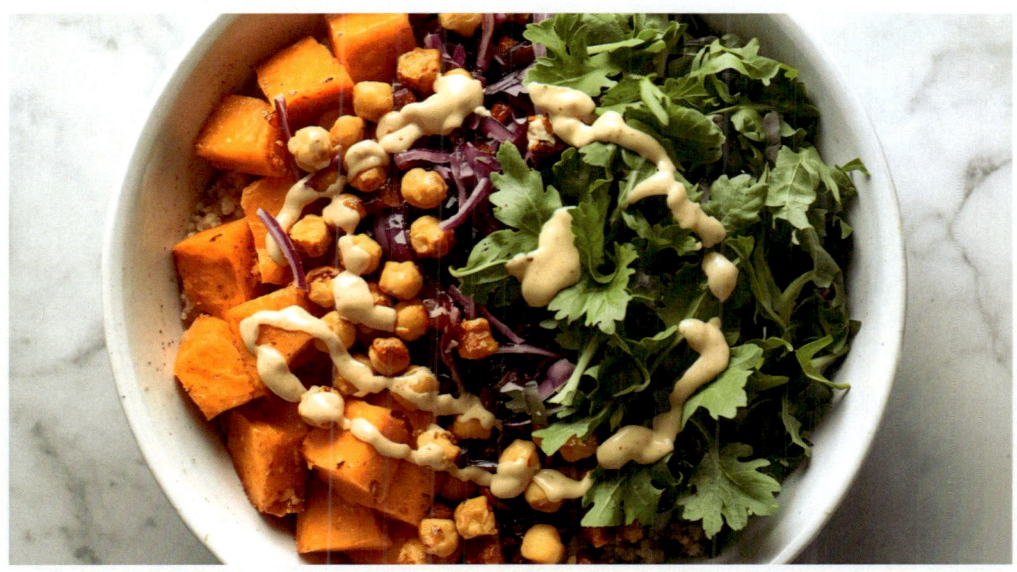

INGREDIENTS: (2 SERVINGS)

- 1 cup quinoa, cooked
- 1 cup roasted sweet potato
- 1 cup purple cabbage, shredded
- 1 cup roasted chickpeas
- 1 cup arugula
- Dressing: 2 tbsp tahini + 1 tbsp lemon juice

INSTRUCTIONS:

- Arrange quinoa, sweet potato, cabbage, chickpeas, and arugula.
- Whisk dressing and drizzle over top.

Mediterranean Abundance Platter

Mantra: "I embody joy and harmony."
Healing Note: Shared meals foster connection.
Ancient Wisdom: Communal feasts symbolized abundance in many traditions.

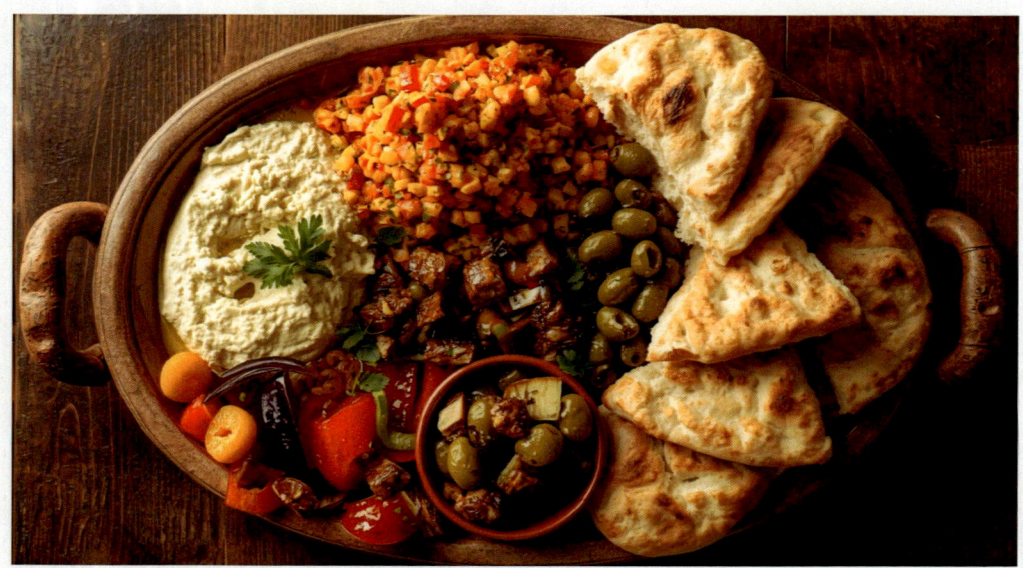

Ingredients: (2 servings)

- ½ cup hummus
- ½ cup tabbouleh
- 1 cup roasted veggies
- ½ cup olives
- Warm pita bread

Instructions:

- Arrange hummus, tabbouleh, veggies, olives, pita on platter.
- Serve as shared meal.

Golden Turmeric Cauliflower Steaks

MANTRA: "I RADIATE GOLDEN ABUNDANCE."
HEALING NOTE: CAULIFLOWER STRENGTHENS DIGESTION; TURMERIC REDUCES INFLAMMATION.
ANCIENT WISDOM: TURMERIC WAS CALLED "THE GOLDEN SPICE OF LIFE" IN AYURVEDA.

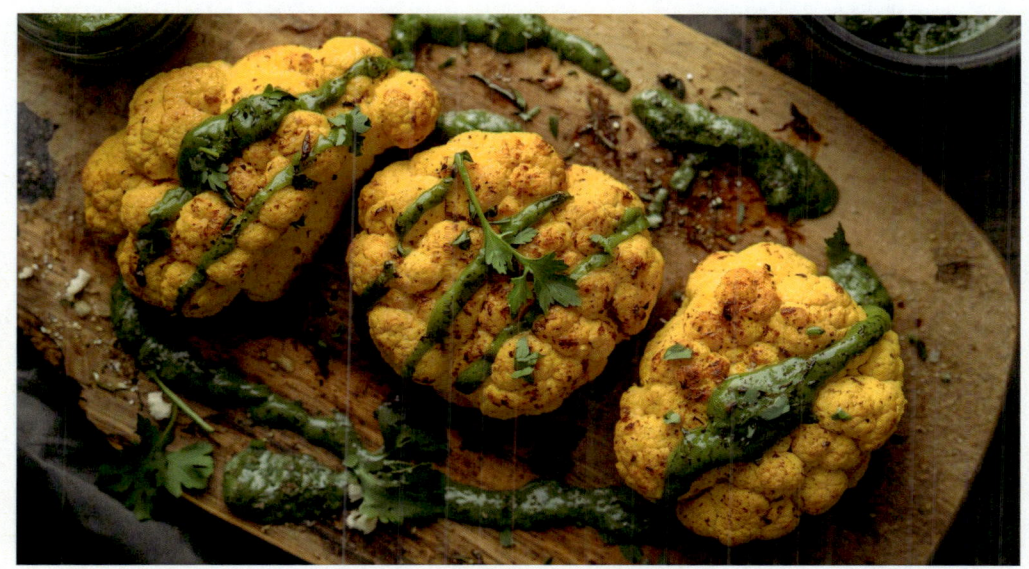

INGREDIENTS: (2 SERVINGS)

- 1 head cauliflower, sliced into 2 "steaks"
- 2 tbsp olive oil
- 1 tsp turmeric
- ½ tsp cumin
- Salt & pepper
- Fresh parsley to garnish

INSTRUCTIONS:

- Preheat oven to 425°F. Place cauliflower steaks on a baking sheet.
- Mix oil, turmeric, cumin, salt & pepper; brush onto cauliflower.
- Roast 25 minutes, flipping once, until golden and tender.
- Garnish with parsley, serve warm.

Roasted Sweet Potato & Pomegranate Bowl

Mantra: "I embody vitality and joy."
Healing Note: Sweet potatoes ground energy; pomegranate boosts renewal.
Ancient Wisdom: Pomegranates were sacred symbols of fertility in Persian culture.

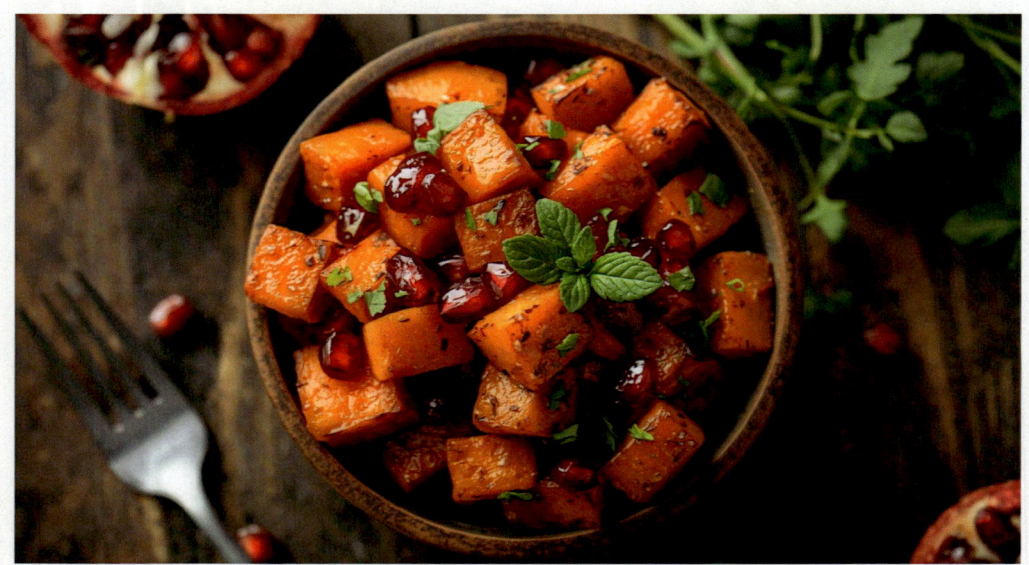

INGREDIENTS: (2 SERVINGS)

- 2 sweet potatoes, cubed
- 1 tbsp olive oil
- 1 cup kale, massaged with lemon juice
- ½ cup pomegranate seeds
- 2 tbsp tahini drizzle

INSTRUCTIONS:

- Toss sweet potatoes with oil, roast at 400°F for 25 minutes.
- Place kale in bowls, top with roasted sweet potatoes.
- Sprinkle pomegranate seeds, drizzle tahini.

Golden Glow Smoothie

MANTRA: "I RADIATE ABUNDANCE AND LIGHT."
HEALING NOTE: TROPICAL FRUITS UPLIFT MOOD.
ANCIENT WISDOM: GOLD-TONED FOODS WERE EATEN FOR PROSPERITY.

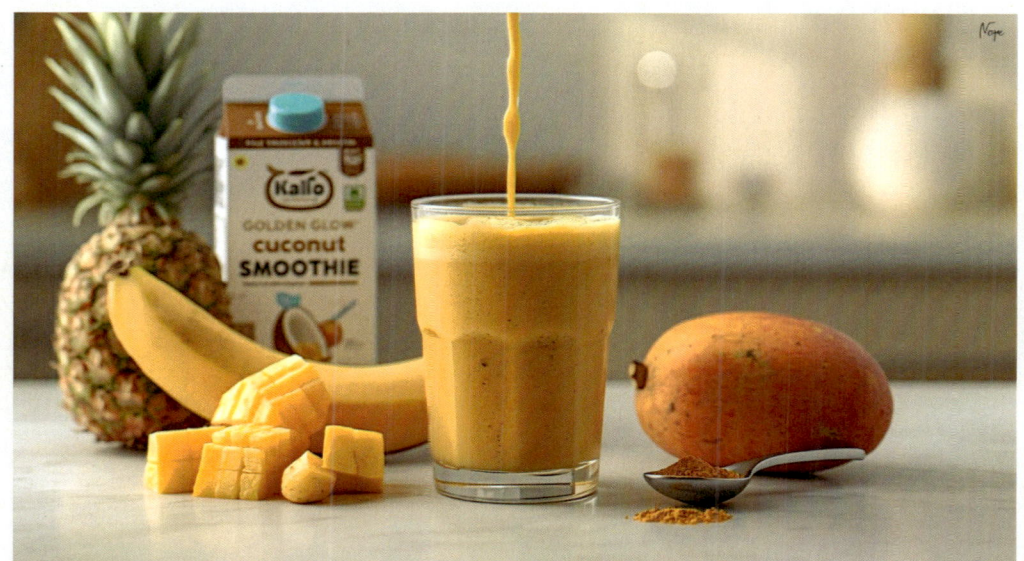

INGREDIENTS: (2 GLASSES)

- 1 cup pineapple
- 1 banana
- 1 cup mango
- 1 cup coconut milk
- ½ tsp turmeric

INSTRUCTIONS:

- Blend all ingredients until smooth.
- Serve chilled.

Cacao Energy Bliss Balls

Mantra: "I energize my body with joy."
Healing Note: Dates give quick natural energy; cacao elevates mood and focus.
Ancient Wisdom: Nuts and seeds have been carried for centuries as symbols of strength and vitality.

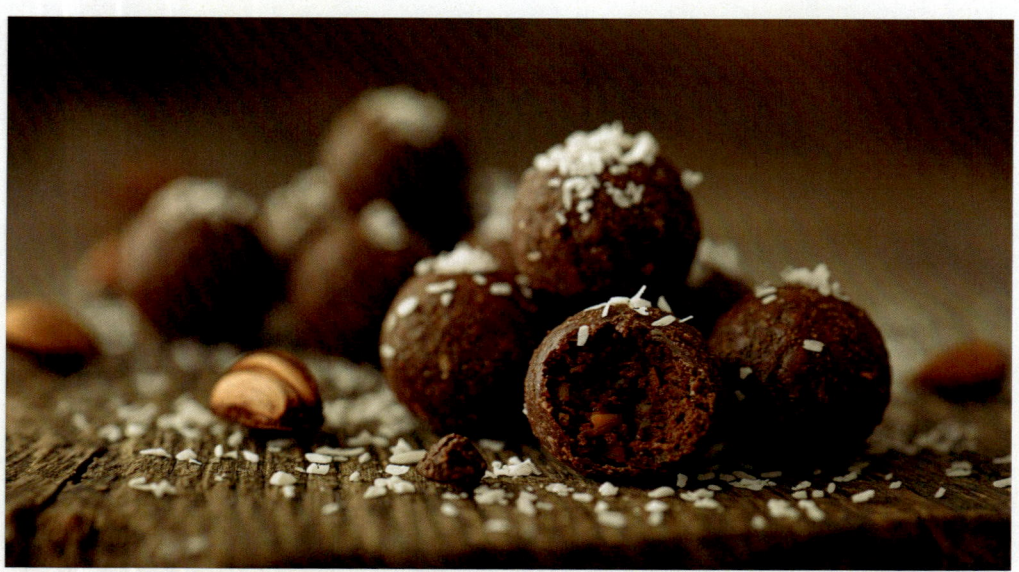

INGREDIENTS: (10-12 Balls)

- 1 cup pitted dates
- ½ cup walnuts or almonds
- ¼ cup raw cacao powder
- 2 tbsp chia or flax seeds
- 1 tsp vanilla extract
- Pinch sea salt
- (Optional) shredded coconut or extra cacao for rolling

INSTRUCTIONS:

- In a food processor, pulse the nuts until finely ground.
- Add dates, cacao, chia/flax, vanilla, and salt. Blend until mixture becomes sticky.
- Scoop about 1 tbsp at a time and roll between your palms to form balls.
- (Optional) Roll balls in shredded coconut or dust with cacao.
- Place on a tray and refrigerate for at least 1 hour before serving.

Berry Bliss Tart

MANTRA: "I EMBODY SWEETNESS AND JOY."
HEALING NOTE: BERRIES ENERGIZE THE HEART.
ANCIENT WISDOM: BERRIES WERE SEEN AS NATURE'S CELEBRATORY GIFTS.

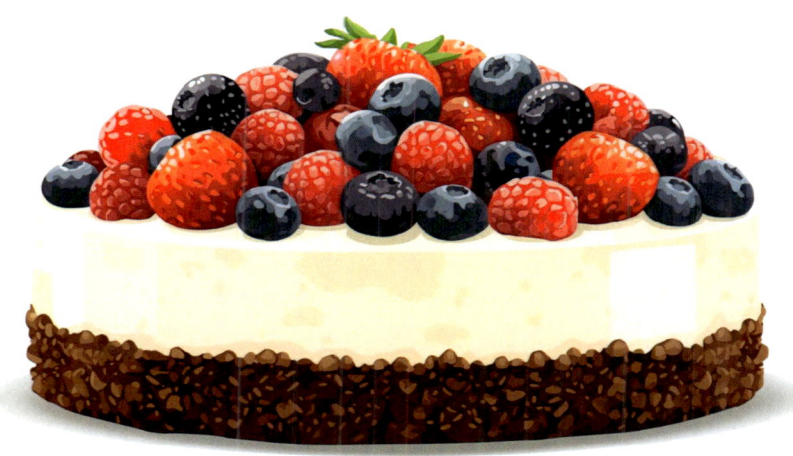

INGREDIENTS: (6 SERVINGS)

Crust: 1 cup almonds + 1 cup dates
Filling: 1 cup coconut cream + 2
tbsp maple syrup
Topping: 1 cup fresh mixed berries

INSTRUCTIONS:

- Blend crust; press into pan.
- Whisk coconut cream + maple; spread into crust.
- Top with berries; chill 2 hrs.

Mango Chia Pudding

Mantra: "I embody joy and sweetness."
Healing Note: Chia hydrates and energizes; mango uplifts mood.
Ancient Wisdom: Mangoes were revered in Vedic tradition as fruit of prosperity and love.

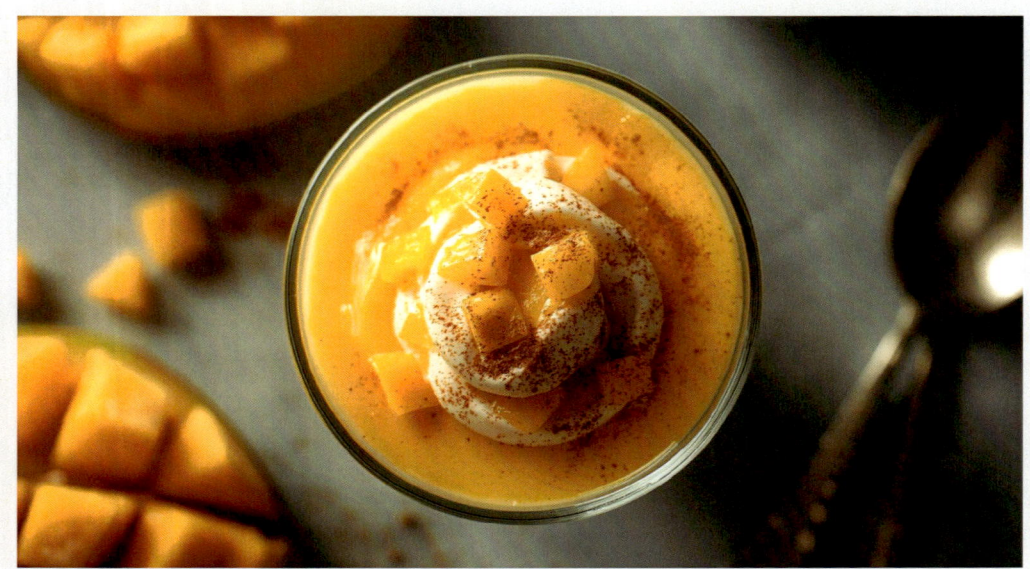

INGREDIENTS: (2 SERVINGS)

- 1 cup almond milk
- 3 tbsp chia seeds
- 1 ripe mango, diced
- 1 tsp maple syrup (optional)
- Pinch of cinnamon

INSTRUCTIONS:

- Stir chia seeds into almond milk; refrigerate 2–3 hours until thick.
- Blend half the mango into puree, fold into chia pudding.
- Top with diced mango and cinnamon.

Cacao Strawberry Celebration Parfait

Mantra: "I celebrate sweetness, connection, and joy."

Healing Note: Strawberries uplift the heart and boost serotonin, while cacao supports circulation, joy, and emotional warmth. This parfait is both grounding and heart-opening — blending nourishment with pleasure to remind you that celebration itself is medicine.

Ancient Wisdom: Cacao was used in sacred rituals by the Aztecs to honor the divine within, while strawberries symbolized love and abundance in Roman feasts. Together, they awaken the heart and remind us to savor life's sweetest moments.

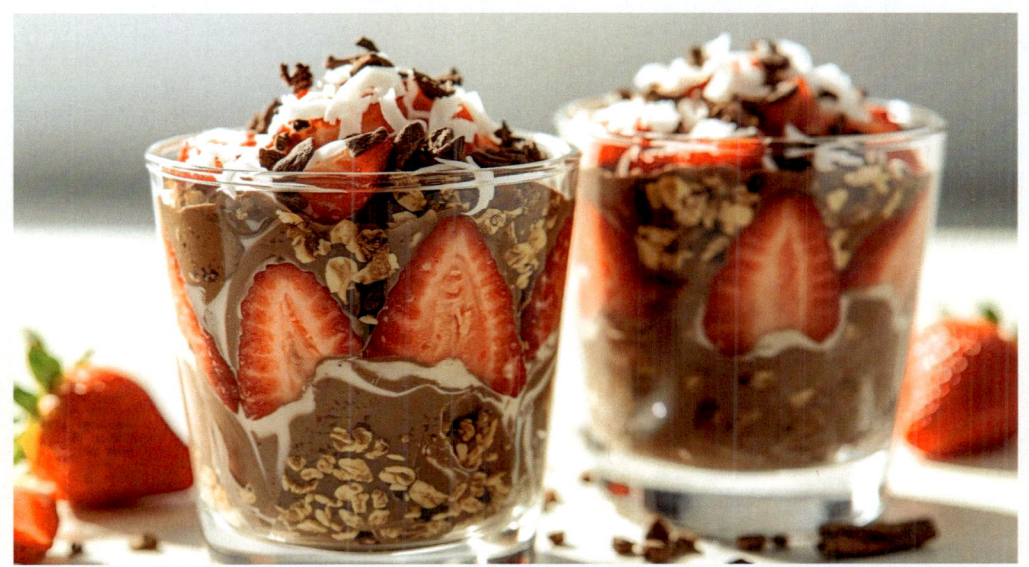

INGREDIENTS: (2 SERVINGS)

- 1 cup coconut yogurt or Greek-style plant yogurt
- 1 tbsp raw cacao powder
- 1–2 tsp maple syrup or honey (to taste)
- 1 tsp vanilla extract
- 1 cup fresh strawberries, sliced
- 2 tbsp granola or crushed nuts (for layering)
- 1 tbsp shredded coconut or cacao nibs (for topping)

INSTRUCTIONS:

- In a small bowl, mix coconut yogurt with cacao powder, vanilla, and maple syrup until creamy and smooth.
- In two glasses or jars, layer ingredients:
- Spoon a layer of cacao yogurt
- Add a layer of strawberries
- Sprinkle with granola or nuts
- Repeat until glasses are full
- Top with shredded coconut or cacao nibs.
- Chill for 15 minutes (optional) before serving for a firmer texture.

FOOD IS MORE THAN WHAT WE EAT—
IT IS HOW WE CHOOSE TO LIVE.
THROUGH THESE RECIPES, YOU'VE
PRACTICED NOURISHMENT AS RITUAL,
GROUNDED IN ANCIENT WISDOM,
AND INFUSED WITH JOY.

Take a quiet moment here to reflect:
Which meal or ritual made me feel most alive?
How has my relationship with food shifted during this
journey?
Where in my life do I feel abundance growing?

Final Mantra: "I am nourished. I am abundant. I am whole."

This is not the end. It is the beginning of embodying joy in
every meal, every moment, and every breath.

TRUEJOY-LIVING  KITCHEN

THANK YOU

"You are the chef of your own transformation.
May this food be your ritual, your healing, and
your joy."
— With love & gratitude,

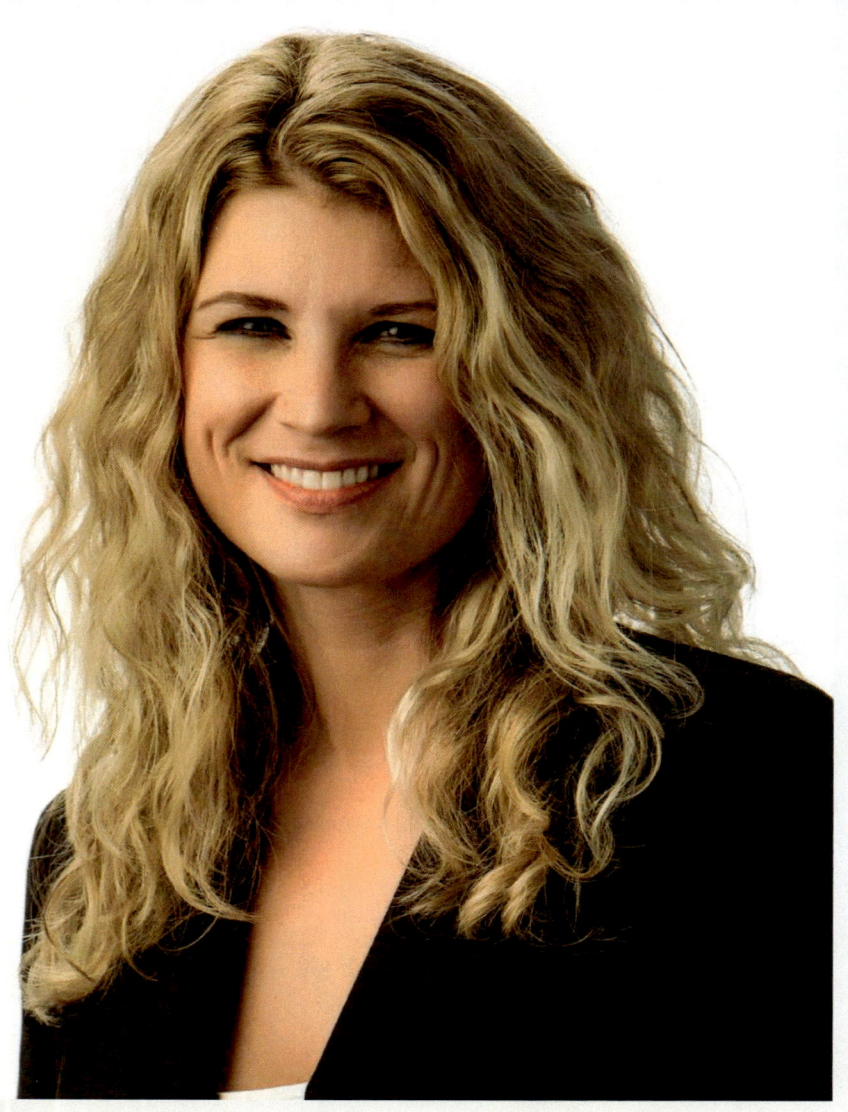

About the Author

Hi, I'm Joy Hafner, the heart behind TrueJoy Living.

I created the Breakthrough Blueprint and the Year of Transformation because I believe that true healing and abundance come from integrating mind, body, and spirit into everyday life.

Food has always been one of my favorite ways to connect with myself and others. Each recipe in this book is designed as a ritual — to ground you, energize you, and remind you that joy is always available, even in the smallest moments.

When I'm not creating recipes or guiding transformation, you'll probably find me barefoot in nature, sipping cacao, or journaling by the ocean.

May these meals nourish you, inspire you, and bring you back home to yourself.

With love,

Joy ✽